Healed

Health & Wellness for the 21st Century

Wisdom, Secrets, and **Fun** Straight from the Leading Edge

"Healed: Health and Wellness for the 21st Century provides the inspiration to live a healthier life by providing spot-on evidence from experts and through the telling of numerous real-life stories of folks overcoming health obstacles. Best of all, the authors teach us how to harness our own brainpower. *Healed* empowers the reader to embrace a healthy lifestyle with a whole food, Mediterranean-style diet, social interaction, and proper and frequent exercise. This excellent read provides compelling evidence that the activity of dancing can provide profound benefits, including that those who dance frequently have a lower risk of dementia! I hope you dance!"

—Donna Hill Howes, RN, MS SVP
Chief Nursing Officer, Sharecare Inc.

"Dr. Robin Miller and her colleague, Dave Kahn, have stepped out of the conventional medical box and provided an innovative approach to healing and being well. They combine leading edge science with some basic key advice to help anyone take charge of their own health in an easy to read format full of interesting patient stories. As a physician-educator, I wish more doctors took Dr. Miller's approach to healing and listening to patients. This book should be required reading for any healthcare professional who wants to expand their ability to both help patients heal, as well as prevent problems. Thanks and keep on dancing, Robin and Dave."

—Kevin Soden, MD, author and medical journalist
*"The Art of Medicine: What Every Doctor
and Patient Should Know"*.
Winner of Emmy, Telly, and International Freddie Awards
Host of Healthline on the Retirement Living Network.

"Everyone and anyone interested in being healthier, happier and living longer must read this book. Dr. Robin Miller combines her vast medical wisdom with her integrative medicine touch to improve everyone's quality and quantity of life. Her co-author Dave Kahn gives great information that is sure to improve everyone's ability to become healthy and fit. Since following their plan I am happier, healthier, have more energy, and get sick much less often. It's a healthy living recipe for all ages!"

—Tanya Altmann, MD, FAAP, pediatrician and author
"What to Feed Your Baby: A Pediatrician's Guide
to the 11 Essential Foods to Guarantee Veggie-Loving,
No-Fuss, Healthy-Eating Kids"

"The ideas Robin and Dave present in this book can be started at any point in the wellness process. Readers can start from wherever they currently are, and by the time they have implemented these ideas they will be well on their way to a healthier, happier life! This book is a must read for anyone wanting to maximize wellness physically, mentally, and emotionally. The authors make it fun to learn and easy to improve life for anyone!"

—Angie Meeker, Pharm.D.
Compounding Pharmacist

"What a detailed, surprising, extremely informative, easy to read book! *Healed* is so chock-full of useful information about our brain, gut, and heart health, that I took notes and now have them on my bulletin board as a reminder of all the great things I can do for my total well-being. Top of the list is sign up for dancing lessons!"

—Jahnna Beecham, editor
National Geographic's Science Encyclopedia

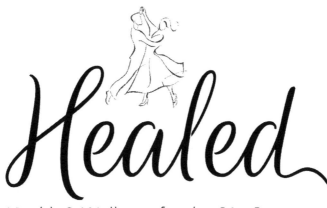

Healed

Health & Wellness for the 21st Century

Wisdom, Secrets, and Fun Straight from the Leading Edge

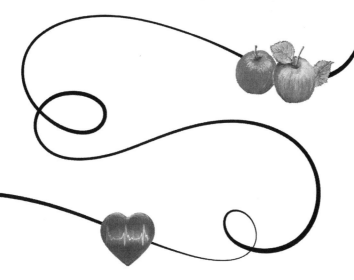

by Robin H. Miller, MD, MHS
& David Es. Kahn, MS, CPT

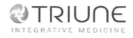

Healed: Health and Wellness for the 21st Century
Wisdom, Secrets, and Fun Straight from the Leading Edge
www.wellhealed.net

ISBN: 978-0-9972030-2-8 (pbk)
ISBN: 978-0-9972030-3-5 (eBook)

Triune Integrative Medicine, LLC
2860 Creekside Circle
Medford, OR 97504
www.TriuneMed.com
(541) 842-9433

Printed in the United States of America

Book cover design by Christy Collins
Book design by Maggie McLaughlin

*The natural healing force in each one of us
is the greatest force in getting well*

—HIPPOCRATES

Acknowledgments

Robin's Acknowledgments: I would like to acknowledge the support and patience of my family, my husband Dr. Peter Adesman and my son's, David and Brian. I am grateful for the advice and support of my friends and colleagues, Becky Nebelsick, Dianne Oceana, Barbara Cecil, Doris Roser, and my pushy trainer, Lynda Sorensen. I am very grateful for the inspiration from the West Coast Swing dance community. Last but certainly not least, a huge thanks and major expression of gratitude to my writing partner, dance partner, teacher, and dear friend, Dave Kahn.

Dave's Acknowledgments: I dedicate this book to my amazing kids, Ben and Amelia, and to all my amazing parents. May the vital information in this book help you to love and live your life all the more. Deepest thanks to my writing partner and dear friend, Robin Miller, without whom I would have no one to bother about when to use whom. Finally, thanks to all my community, my huge concatenation of friends, in West Coast Swing. You make life worth living.

Our thanks to Maggie McLaughlin for her editing expertise, Christy Collins for designing our cover, and Jennifer Margulis, Tess Minnick and Val Blazer for their help and guidance.

Contents

INTRODUCTION   xiii

PART I: THE BASICS   1

1   On Finding a Partner in Wellness   3

2   The Heart   7

3   The Gut   15

4   The Brain   27

PART II: WHAT'S NEW?   43

5   Longevity   45

6   Depression   51

7   Trust Your Gut and Take Care of It   65

8   Fun Foods That You Didn't Know Were Healthy   71

9   What Women Want When it Comes to Sex   85

PART III: THE UNDIET (AKA THE TEID DIET)   95

10 I Was Too Fat . . .   97

PART IV: DANCE LIKE YOUR LIFE DEPENDS ON IT . . .   115

11 Brain-Power   121

12 Finally! A Program Just for You   129

13 Lower Your Blood Pressure   135

14 Finding the Right Balance—Literally   139

15   Osteoporosis   145

16   Dance for Recovery   149

17   Social Anxiety? Not Any More!   153

18   Breaking Good   161

19   No Paining—Yes Gaining (On Mental Health and Depression)   161

20   Soaring with The Eagles   171

AFTERWARD   **177**

Letter   179

Cheat Sheet   181

REFERENCES

Appendix A   Dance Conventions   183

Appendix B   End Notes   187

Appendix C   Sources   191

Appendix D   Index   205

Introduction

I **HAVE BEEN IN** medical practice for over 30 years. I am a general Internist who started by doing research for the first ten years of my career, and then practiced conventional medicine at a medical clinic in Oregon. Ten years ago, I left mainstream medicine to become an Integrative medicine physician. I gave up the ten-minute patient visits for longer ones in order to practice the kind of patient focused medicine I had dreamed of doing when I first went to medical school. Over the years in my varied career, I have picked up quite a few pearls of wisdom along with a hunger to find more ways to help my patients. I have been frustrated by the lack of options available when it comes to conventional medicine. Don't get me wrong. There are amazing treatments and therapies available these days that have allowed our lifespan to increase. However, often I find I cannot help people as much as I would like because I run out of tools and possibilities.

That's fueled my search to step out of the box (actually to sometimes get rid of the box altogether) and find new, innovative ways to help people to heal and be well. Sometimes it requires going back to basics, and other times I have ventured into the wild world of new science, such as the exploding field of genetics and microbiology. Over the years, I have learned so much and found so many relatively simple ways to help patients that I realized it was time to share these ideas and suggestions.

That is how *Healed* was born.

With the help of a very smart and fun colleague, Dave Kahn, I bring you this book. It will take you through the basics of what you need to know to promote your own health, and then together we will bring you to the leading edge of new therapies to treat common conditions such as depression, obesity, cancer and Alzheimer's and Parkinson's disease. Often what seems new is in reality, really old. Some solutions actually go way back to the beginning of Western medicine. Others are just starting to revolutionize care. Finally, I know it sounds too good to be true, but it isn't: we'll introduce you to a form of exercise that is fun, exciting and will help improve just about whatever ails you.

HOW TO READ THIS BOOK

You can read this book from start to finish, but you do not have to go in order. We do think you will enjoy it in its entirety. It is meant to be read actively! So take notes, underline, highlight, and dog-ear the pages!

We have provided you with a "cheat sheet" at the end of the book that will help you to discuss potential tests and treatments with your doctor that are not yet part of mainstream medicine. This will make it easier to initiate the discussion and organize your thoughts.

PART I
THE BASICS

INTRODUCTION

There are many systems in the body I could discuss. However, I have chosen three I feel are most important and are major concerns for the patients I care for. These include the heart, the gut and the brain. We will be getting to many of the other systems in Parts II and IV. But first, you need to find a partner in your care.

1 ON FINDING A PARTNER IN WELLNESS

THE STORY

Many years ago during my residency, I treated a patient in the emergency room, and soon admitted her. Jane had recently had a baby. After the baby was born, Jane developed severe abdominal pain and was diagnosed with appendicitis. Her appendix was removed, but as it turns out, it was normal. The pain got worse. Her doctors decided she was a drug seeker, someone who invents symptoms just to get pain meds.

I spent a lot of time speaking with Jane (a less-traditional approach back then). I learned in addition to taking birth control pills, she wanted to lose her baby weight and had basically stopped eating.

That evening, I went to the library and started researching. It took me awhile, but I figured it out. I raced to her room that night and had her urinate in a cup. I put the cup in the window and waited until morning. Sure enough, on morning rounds, just as the attending physician was getting ready to kick her out of the hospital, I pointed to the urine in the window. The sunlight had turned it a deep purple. What she had was acute intermittent porphyria, a rare disease that occurs in people who are missing a particular enzyme. When patients with this problem diet by fasting and/or are exposed to certain type of anesthesia or take estrogen, the system is stressed and a buildup of a chemical occurs in their blood and urine and causes abdominal pain. Jane had all three triggers.

Experts and Evidence

In medical school, one of the first things I learned was if you listen closely, 99 percent of the time patients will tell you what's wrong with them. But doctors these days are busy—so busy many practice what I call "McDonald's medicine," attempting to diagnose and treat patients in ten minutes or less. It is imperative to find a doctor who listens, since, according to the Centers for Disease Control and Prevention, 75 percent of disease is related to lifestyle choices. It is also critical to find a doctor who's interested in helping you address unhealthy habits.

When I speak to groups of people about this, invariably many will come up to me afterwards and say what I am suggesting is impossible. However, there is a growing field of medicine spreading throughout the country: Integrative medicine. This is what I practice. Integrative medicine is focused on the *patient.* (What a concept!) The provider forms a partnership with the patient to promote wellness. The goal is to address the whole patient: mind, body and spirit. In doing so, the patient will become healthy and well, and disease will be prevented. Conversely, most of medicine these days is disease-oriented. A patient presents with a problem, and that problem is treated. There is little time spent looking at the whole picture and getting at the root of the problem. Integrative medicine practitioners will find ways to help patients heal on their own. For example, when you break a bone, the orthopedic surgeon sets the bone, but your body heals the fracture. When you have a bacterial infection, an antibiotic will decrease the number of bacteria in your body to allow your white blood cells to kill them.

These concepts can be applied to healing in general. It requires a physician who is willing to listen and take the time to explain and educate patients. Fortunately, a fellowship offered by Dr. Andrew Weil at the University of Arizona has been training practitioners for the last 16 years. I am one of his graduates. Through his program and website you can find a doctor near you. Find an Integrative Health Care Provider at https://integrativemedicine.arizona.edu/alumni.html

Now that you know how to find a provider who will listen, I am going to give you some ideas on how to make the most of your visit with any doctor.

BE ORGANIZED

Most regular doctors will only admit privately that they freak out when patients bring in a list. I welcome it. I appreciate when patients have been able to organize their thoughts before they come in to see me. It makes my job much easier—just keep the list to one page. There is a computer app that will help you organize your thoughts. You will find it online or on your phone: AskMD. It will help you record your symptoms in order of importance and give your doctor an excellent printout, along with likely causes.

BE OPEN

If you are seeing someone to get their opinion and ideas about how to improve your health, you will need to leave your own theories and preconceived notions at the door. This will help to optimize your visits. I have had many people come in with ideas that have absolutely no scientific basis regarding what will help them. They refuse to listen to reason. Those are patients who don't come back to see me and probably will not be helped by anyone. There was one woman who thought that bacteria in her colon were dangerous to her body. She wanted me, and her gastroenterologist, to wipe them all out. That would be impossible, and it would literally kill her since we need bacteria (as you will see when we discuss the gut) to live. There was yet another woman who was profoundly hypothyroid and hypertensive who was convinced that dandelion root and iodine were the answers to her problems. She came to see me so I would confirm that.

I did not agree. She needed medication to control her thyroid and her blood pressure. She never came back to see me again. She ended up dying from not properly treating her condition.

BE HONEST

Tell your doctor about your symptoms, concerns and fears. I saw a young man many years ago, before I started my Integrative medicine practice. I was working in urgent care. He wanted opioid pain medications for limb pain. I started questioning him, and found out what was really going on was that his wife was leaving him, and he was devastated. I did not give him the pain medication. I gave him a referral to a therapist. Many years later, once I started my practice, I saw him at a Relay for Life event. He thanked me and told me the night he came to see me in urgent care, he had planned on killing himself, and he was going to do it with the pain medication. He took my advice and got help. He told me his life had turned around, and then he introduced me to his lovely new wife and their beautiful baby.

BE READY TO CHANGE

I can give you all the advice in the world, but if you are not willing to change, nothing will change. We know at least 75 percent of disease is due to unhealthy lifestyle choices.[1] If you are willing to improve yours, you will increase your chances of healing. If not, you won't. This is a very simple concept that is so incredibly hard for most of us to grasp. I have a patient whom I have cared for over the last ten years. I always went through the same drill with her regarding healthy eating and exercise. She suffered from arthritis pain in her knees and back and was always mildly depressed. One day, she decided to follow the lifestyle changes we had discussed. (It had taken about five years for the concept to sink in.) Once she changed her eating and exercise habits, she lost weight; her knees improved and so did her mood. For her, it was nothing short of a miracle. Sometimes it takes a while for the message to get through. I am so glad it did for her, and I keep hoping it will for others, especially after reading this book.

2 THE HEART

THE STORY
Joan was a 68-year-old woman with diabetes and high blood pressure. One evening she experienced intense nausea, heartburn and neck pressure as well as a sense of impending doom. She drove herself to the emergency room, where she was asked to take a seat. She waited quietly for three hours, during which time her condition deteriorated. When doctors finally got to her, she was clammy and weak and her blood pressure had dropped precipitously. She eventually recovered, but she suffered a heart attack with permanent heart damage that would likely have been avoided if she had recognized the symptoms and responded appropriately—by calling an ambulance and demanding assistance.

Experts and Evidence

The number-one killer of men and women is heart disease. According to the Centers for Disease Control, there are around 610,000 deaths due to heart disease every year in the United States alone.

That is equivalent to one out of every four deaths. There are many public service announcements and a lot of educational materials circulated to help Americans understand how to recognize and prevent heart disease. Unfortunately, many people still don't get it. In 2005, a large study found only 31 percent of the respondents could identify the five major warning signs of a heart attack.[1] This is particularly pertinent to women and those caring for women, since for them the signs of heart attack can be more subtle.

THE WARNING SIGNS OF A HEART ATTACK

CHEST PAIN

This can be severe, like a truck or an elephant sitting on the chest. In women especially, it can be as mild as discomfort or indigestion. I have had a couple of female patients who felt a vague chest pain or ache that was hard for them to describe. One had it on the left and the other in the middle. Neither found relief with antacids or acid blocker medications. It made them anxious, but it was not a panic attack. Panic attacks go away within minutes, and this discomfort did not. That should be a clue it is something more ominous than heartburn.

PAIN IN THE ARMS AND SHOULDER

This does not always occur. When it does happen, many people dismiss it, thinking they may have slept wrong or lifted something heavy. The pain is usually more of an ache rather than soreness. It is often described as an overwhelming feeling of weakness, and in many it will occur while exercising.

PAIN IN THE JAW, NECK OR BACK

I have had a couple of women patients who only complained of jaw pain while they were having a heart attack. Both went to the dentist thinking it was a toothache. What they failed to mention to the dentists were the symptoms they did not want to acknowledge to themselves: accompanying fatigue and total body weakness that were also present with the pain. This should have been a tip-off it was more than just a toothache.

SHORTNESS OF BREATH

When the onset is unexplained, it should arouse concern. Continued shortness of breath accompanied by fatigue or discomfort should set off alarm bells that the heart is in jeopardy. In addition, patients may experience overwhelming fatigue, nausea, sweating, anxiety or uneasiness and a sense of impending doom.

FEELING DIZZY OR LIGHTHEADED

I had a patient who experienced severe nausea and vomiting and dizziness along with the above symptoms. She was sure she had food poisoning. Rather than get better after her violent spells, she continued to get weaker until she finally collapsed and was sent to the ER.

DON'T WAIT

If you have any of the above symptoms, listen to your body and trust your gut. Intuition is a powerful thing. If you think something serious is going on, you are probably correct. Call 911 immediately. Time is of the essence. While waiting for the ambulance chew a 325 mg aspirin. That will help thin the blood and potentially improve the blocked artery causing the pain.

EVALUATE YOUR RISK

There are a variety of risk factors that can increase the chances of having a heart attack. Some are genetic and others are very preventable. The classic genetic factors that put you at risk for hardening of the arteries and heart attack include:

- ☑ A family history of heart disease in a first-degree relative (mother, father, sister or brother).
- ☑ Increasing age ups the risk for heart disease.
- ☑ Men are at higher risk at first; women catch up after menopause.
- ☑ High cholesterol or increased lipids or fats in the blood. (These tend to be hereditary.)
- ☑ High blood pressure (can be hereditary as well).

FACTORS YOU CAN CHANGE INCLUDE:

- ☑ Obesity
- ☑ A sedentary lifestyle
- ☑ Tobacco use
- ☑ Diabetes
- ☑ Stress
- ☑ Depression
- ☑ Loneliness
- ☑ History of autoimmune disease
- ☑ TMAO (Trimethylamine N-oxide—*more on this shortly*)

WHAT CAN YOU DO?

Obviously, you cannot prevent aging or change your genetics. But there are things you can control. First things first: become informed. Make sure to have your blood pressure checked at least yearly as well as your cholesterol and fasting blood sugar. Have your weight checked. Many people who are overweight or obese do not recognize (or admit) they have an issue. Extra poundage adds extra risk for diabetes, heart disease, stroke, certain cancers and a variety of other problems. If you would like an actual number that gives you your risk, there is an app for that! It is free. Go to ASCVD Risk Estimator. It will ask for your age, gender, race, systolic blood pressure, treatment for high blood pressure and it will ask if you are a smoker and/or a diabetic. It will also ask for your total cholesterol and HDL cholesterol. These values you get from a simple blood test done by your doctor, called a lipid panel.

CHECK YOUR CHOLESTEROL

When it comes to measuring cholesterol, I usually recommend a one-time blood test that measures the actual cholesterol particles. This is a test most physicians do not do routinely, but I find it to be very helpful. It is called the NMR lipoprofile study. It will show the actual value of your LDL or "bad cholesterol." The usual lipid profile calculates the bad or LDL cholesterol using an equation: LDL cholesterol = Total Cholesterol − HDL (the good cholesterol) − Triglycerides/5.

This test does not give a view of the whole picture. There are other particles that may help predict the risk for heart disease. There are different types of LDL. They are the large type particles which are big and fluffy and not as toxic as the small particle type, which are dense and can eat away at arteries and cause plaque. There are two types of HDL cholesterol: type 2, which is large and protective, and type 3, which is not as protective.

The NMR test is far more helpful, in my opinion, to see if cholesterol levels really need to be treated with medication. I am much more likely to recommend a cholesterol lowering drug to a patient who presents with small dense LDL particles and low HDL 2 levels. In addition, because everything is measured in this test, I am able to see what a patient's triglyceride levels look like when they are non-fasting. This can be very helpful because high triglycerides in general (fasting or not) can increase the risk for an inflamed pancreas. If the test is done fasting, there is a measure that will show an increased risk for insulin resistance or metabolic syndrome. Metabolic syndrome is defined by a group of problems, including high blood pressure, increased blood sugar, and fat around the middle leading to an increased risk for heart disease.

CHECK YOUR BLOOD PRESSURE

If you are found to have high blood pressure in the doctor's office, start checking your blood pressure at home. I have many patients who only have high blood pressure in my office, but it is because I either make them nervous or just being in a doctor's office makes them nervous and causes a momentary blood pressure rise. They do not need to be on medication. If there is any question as to what time of day their blood pressure is elevated, I use a 24–hour blood pressure monitor they wear at home. It records blood pressures throughout the day. This has been enormously helpful for them. Ask your doctor about one of these devices if you think you may have variable blood pressures related to stressful situations.

A great example of unusual blood pressure elevations due to stress is a nurse whom I take care of. She became alarmed when someone at work checked her blood pressure and it was sky-high. She wondered if she needed medication. The 24-hour monitor showed that her blood pressure was only high at work when she was assigned to a particular doctor. She made some changes at work and is no longer working with that particular person. Now no more high blood pressure—problem solved!

QUIT SMOKING

Tobacco use is a major risk factor for heart disease and stroke and needs to be stopped; preferably never started. The moment you stop, your risk diminishes. Yes, it is very hard to quit smoking, but millions have done it. Today there are many things available to help. There are nicotine patches, gums and inhalers, and there are even medications for extreme cases. There are smoking cessation groups. Hypnosis and acupuncture help as well. If you are still smoking, make it a priority to free yourself and save your body from this horribly dangerous (and expensive) habit.

GET MOVING

Along the lines of smoking, sitting all day can be just as bad and is considered the "new smoking." [2] It can be just as deleterious to your heart and overall health! The moment you start moving on a regular basis, your health improves. A small pedal bike that can be placed under a desk has been found to help with weight loss and make exercise possible while even sitting at a desk.

ADOPT A HEALTHY LIFESTYLE

Diabetes can destroy your body. The major cause for type 2 diabetes is obesity. Exercise, a healthy diet and general movement throughout the day can all help improve blood sugar and prevent diabetes. Later on, we will present suggestions for healthy eating and exercise that will get you feeling healthier and even looking better. These same suggestions will help with loneliness, stress and depression, all of which can contribute to the development of heart disease. As far as autoimmune disease goes, an anti-inflammatory diet known as the

Mediterranean diet can help, and that is what we will be discussing in Chapter 7.

TMAO

What about TMAO (mentioned in our risk-factor list)? What is it? It stands for trimethylamine N-oxide, something you don't want in your body. Recently, researchers from the Cleveland Clinic have identified it as a potent risk factor for heart disease and stroke. They have found through multiple studies when we eat foods high in L-carnitine and choline, the organisms in our gut metabolize them into trimethylamine N-oxide (TMAO). This chemical causes inflammation in our blood vessels that leads to narrowing and lack of blood flow, which ultimately can lead to heart attack and stroke. Red meat is particularly high in L-carnitine. Farm-raised fish and egg yolks are high in choline. This discovery is relatively recent and recommendations in the future will be forthcoming. In the meantime, I have been recommending my patients have a fasting TMAO level done. This is available through the Cleveland Heart Lab. If levels are over 6.2 mM (this unit is a laboratory measure of TMAO concentration in the blood and stands for micromoles), I recommend they eliminate or decrease the amount of red meat they eat. In general, I urge my patients to eat only wild-caught fish. As far as egg yolks go, those with high TMAO levels should probably limit their consumption and switch to egg whites. If elevated TMAO is a problem, food such as grape seed extract, extra virgin olive oil and (believe it or not!) Guinness Stout can lower levels.

SUMMING UP YOUR HEART

There is constant chatter regarding the risk factors for heart attack and heart disease. I am not sure why the message is not being received. I think one of the reasons is that, despite knowing the signs, we tend to think it will not happen to us. Women in particular ignore the symptoms. We keep on going, doing what we do, which is usually taking care of everyone else first before taking care of ourselves. But remember you cannot take care of anyone if you are not here.

Joan, the patient who sat in the ER waiting room and proceeded to have a heart attack, never heeded that advice. Her diabetes worsened, she was too busy to exercise and she was too busy to shop for healthy foods. Three years after her heart attack, she died of a stroke. That is why understanding your risks, doing something to decrease them and finding a lifestyle that will maximize your health is so important. Please take this advice to heart; I wish Joan had.

3 THE GUT

WHEN LIFE TURNS topsy-turvy, our digestive system sometimes follows suit. But for people with irritable bowel syndrome (IBS), there's no such thing as smooth sailing. Any day, any moment might bring abdominal discomfort, cramps, and bouts of diarrhea, constipation, or all of these symptoms, along with gas and bloating. It is *not* a fun ride. The key to calming the intestinal seas is sussing out what's causing the problem. Once you round that buoy, relief is in sight.

It's hard to know how many people have IBS since many cases go undiagnosed, but one survey found about 14 percent of Americans suffer from it—more than 43 million people! [1] Twice as many women have it as men, and people ages 25 to 54 are most vulnerable.

The triggers can be variable. Certain foods such as chocolate, wheat and vegetables can increase the symptoms. Stress also plays a significant role.

But not all digestive problems that seem like IBS actually are. In fact, IBS is what we call a diagnosis of exclusion, or **I Be S**tumped. When all other likely possibilities have been ruled out, it's likely IBS.

To illustrate the difficulty of the IBS diagnosis, I give you the Tales of Four Women, all with "gut-wrenching" difficulties. Only two actually had IBS, but all four got major relief once they found the right treatment. Read on.

THE STORIES:

BETH

Beth, a young woman of 26, had suffered her whole life with severe abdominal pain that came and went. She also complained of horrible gas that was particularly smelly.

On talking with Beth, it seemed her symptoms were worse after she ate dairy products and fruit. I sent her to a gastroenterologist to get two different breath tests. The first test, a hydrogen breath test, looked at her ability to digest dairy. She was given a milk preparation to drink, and then she blew into special bags every 20 minutes for three hours. The bags were analyzed for the presence of hydrogen and methane. She had high levels of both, which pointed to lactose intolerance (a deficiency of lactase, the enzyme that digests milk sugars) and an overgrowth in the small intestine of a type of bacteria that produces methane. We treated her with antibiotics and asked her to cut out dairy and fruit in an effort to starve the methane-producing bacteria in her gut. It worked and she improved, but she still wasn't "right."

Next she had a fructose tolerance test to test her ability to digest fruit. The same procedure was repeated, this time after she drank a fructose drink. Sure enough, she was found to also have fructose intolerance. The fructose drink stirred up her old symptoms again, so we gave her another course of antibiotics to treat the bacterial overgrowth. Finally, her symptoms have resolved after a lifetime of suffering. And now she knows what foods to avoid so they don't come back.

Beth had food intolerances and bacterial overgrowth, but not true IBS, since her symptoms resolved once the causes were eradicated.

ANNA

Anna is a 50-year-old woman who came to see me for a new patient physical. She told me she was healthy, but as we talked, I discovered she suffered from abdominal discomfort she hadn't thought to mention because she'd simply gotten used to having it. She had suffered intermittent bouts of diarrhea and also low-level fatigue for years.

As part of her evaluation, I did a blood test to check for celiac disease. This is an inflammatory condition of the small intestine that results from an allergy to gluten. Her test was markedly positive. In addition, all her vitamin levels were low. This wasn't a surprise, since celiac disease compromises the ability of the gastrointestinal tract to absorb vitamins from food.

The treatment for her was to cut out gluten from her diet. This means avoiding not only the obvious things like most bread, pasta, cereal, crackers and cookies, but also a whole host of other food products, including most beer, baked goods, candy, french fries, gravy, imitation seafood, salad dressings, some sauces (including soy sauce), seasoned rice mixes, and some soups and seasoned snack foods, to name many but not all. Gluten is even found in some cosmetics!

Anna has been very good at avoiding these foods and is doing well. She no longer has abdominal discomfort and her energy level has skyrocketed. She is a bit upset, however; now that she is absorbing nutrients from food properly, she has gained ten pounds!

Like Beth, Anna didn't have IBS. Her celiac disease was the problem, and a change of diet was the solution.

CAROL

Carol had suffered with irritable bowel symptoms her whole life. But breath tests and a colonoscopy turned up nothing. During the course of her evaluation, Carol shared her personal history with me—and it was not pretty.

She grew up in a dysfunctional family and had been molested and physically and emotionally abused. She left home at 15. She lived on the streets for some time and had been raped and beaten. Miraculously, she was able to get her life together. She now has a thriving business and a wonderful family. However, she had IBS symptoms that were disabling.

I referred her to a psychologist for eye movement desensitization reprocessing (EMDR) therapy. This technique is most often used to treat people with post-traumatic stress disorder, but it's also useful for anyone who's lived through a traumatic stress of any sort and is suffering from physical symptoms. In this therapy, a specially trained psychologist distracts your brain, either by having you follow her finger with your eyes or by making tapping or other sounds, while you conjure a disturbing memory from your past. Soon the power of those bad memories is significantly reduced. (Read more about EMDR in Chapter 6.) Carol had four treatments and her symptoms completely resolved.

GAIL

Gail, who is 55, had lived her whole life with a low level of depression and abdominal symptoms. As part of her evaluation, I did a test that checked for mutations in a gene that helps process folic acid, a B vitamin.

When people have one or more mutations of a particular gene, called MTHFR (methylenetetrahydrofolate reductase), they can't process folic acid efficiently—and they may feel it in their gut since folic acid plays a role in keeping the gut happy. MTHFR *is* good when it's working properly in the body; it helps turn folic acid into L-methylfolate, an active form of the vitamin. The body needs this active form to make the "feel-good" hormones serotonin, dopamine and norepinephrine. You probably think of serotonin as a brain chemical. But—surprise!—the gastrointestinal system is lined with cells that look like brain cells, and they secrete serotonin, too.

Gail had two mutations on her MTHFR gene. I prescribed supplements of L-methylfolate at a high dose and her IBS symptoms went away. Her depression resolved as well! (Read more about L-methylfolate in Chapter 6.)

Experts and Evidence

THE FOODS THAT AIL US: ALLERGIES ALL AROUND

As you discovered above, many digestive problems that seem like IBS actually stem from food intolerance. If you have food intolerance, you're lucky in one sense because your symptoms will most likely disappear after you cut the problem foods out of your diet. Below are some of the most common intolerances.

LACTOSE INTOLERANCE

Got milk? If you do and you're lactose intolerant, you probably also have diarrhea, bloating, belly pain and maybe even nausea.

Lactose intolerance is caused by a deficiency of the enzyme lactase. Produced by the small intestine, it helps the body digest lactose, a sugar found in milk and other dairy products. (Yes, milk contains natural sugars, even before you add the chocolate syrup.)

You might think you're either born lactose intolerant or not, but in fact, lactase deficiency develops over time and becomes more common with age. It can also occur after chemotherapy for cancer. People with Inflammatory bowel disease (IBD) are also at increased risk.

There are two ways to diagnose the condition. The easiest way is to avoid milk products and see if your digestive problems go away.

The other is to take the same breath test Beth took: first you consume a dairy drink, and then you breathe into a special bag over the course of several hours. If the hydrogen level in your breath is high, you have lactase deficiency and are therefore lactose intolerant.

Most people who are lactose intolerant can tolerate a little bit of lactose, and some can tolerate yogurt with active cultures (thanks to the lactase-producing "cultures," or bacteria) and/or hard cheeses. Your tolerance depends on how much or how little lactase your body produces. Taking an enzyme supplement such as Lactaid or Similase can help you digest dairy more easily. Probiotics, including the extra-strong product VSL#3 (which should be used only under the supervision of the doctor treating you for IBS) can also aid digestion.

FRUCTOSE INTOLERANCE

An apple a day might help keep the doctor away, but not for someone with fructose intolerance, also known as fructose malabsorption. Some studies suggest it's a common cause of irritable bowel symptoms.[2]

Can someone really be intolerant of fruit? Unfortunately, yes, as Beth's story also illustrated. People with fructose malabsorption have trouble digesting the sugar fructose, found in fruit and anything made with high fructose corn syrup. When these people eat fruit, the sugar is not fully absorbed in their small intestine, so it makes its way to the large intestine—also known as the bowel—where it doesn't belong. There it can wreak havoc, causing problems with gas, bloating, pain and more.

Fructose intolerance can be diagnosed with another type of hydrogen breath test (very similar to the lactose intolerance test). You'll be given a fructose drink and then you'll blow into a bag every 15 minutes for several hours. If you have a lot of hydrogen in your breath, the test is positive.

The easy treatment is to avoid fructose. You would think that would mean avoiding all fruit. Luckily, berries have very low amounts of fructose, so they are generally okay to eat. But other fruits and foods with high fructose corn syrup will cause problems.

GLUTEN INTOLERANCE

If you've never noticed the sprouting of gluten-free products on grocery store shelves, you will now. It seems every other person we meet is going gluten-free. Contrary to popular belief, cutting out gluten will not help you lose weight, not any more than cutting out simple carbs in general will. So if weight loss is your objective, you might as well embrace gluten again. But some people do have gluten intolerance (not to be confused with celiac disease). They may experience IBS-type symptoms after eating wheat, rye, barley or other gluten-containing foods. For people with this intolerance, avoiding gluten will relieve their symptoms. However, if they eat some gluten on occasion, it won't hurt them, in contrast to people with celiac disease, who shouldn't consume any gluten ever.

If you test negative for celiac disease, that doesn't mean you don't have gluten intolerance. Unfortunately, there is no definitive test for gluten intolerance. The best way to know if you have it is to avoid gluten for 30 days and see if your symptoms improve. (Look back at Anna's story for a partial list of foods that contain gluten.)

CELIAC DISEASE

We told you Anna's story earlier in this chapter. She was diagnosed with celiac disease, which is an autoimmune disease that results in gluten intolerance. You might say it's the "it" disease of the century. It turns out about 1 in 140 Americans has celiac disease! [3] If you do, your body attacks the cells of the small intestine when it is exposed to gluten. The result is poor absorption of nutrients, leading to nutritional deficiencies.

Some people have very few symptoms. Others experience diarrhea or constipation, bloating, vitamin D deficiency, itchy skin rashes and other autoimmune problems such as thyroiditis (inflammation of the thyroid gland). If celiac disease goes untreated, it can also cause a host of difficult or even life-threatening symptoms. These include fatigue, bone or joint pain, osteoporosis, depression, canker sores, tingling in the hands or feet, missed menstrual periods and

even infertility or frequent miscarriages. It can also result in mal-
nutrition, anemia, and increase the risk for certain cancers such as
lymphoma.[4]

Celiac disease is diagnosed by a blood test and confirmed by a
small bowel biopsy, which can be done with upper endoscopy by
a gastroenterologist. (In this test, the doctor places a long, flexible
tube with a camera at its tip down your esophagus.)

The treatment is relatively simple: completely avoid gluten. Since
the awareness of celiac disease has increased, so has the availability
of gluten-free products.

A FINAL WORD ABOUT FOOD ALLERGIES

Why do so many people have food sensitivities today? There are
many theories. One theory—and it's just that, an unproven theory,
tested only in animals such as pigs and sheep—holds that genetically
modified foods in our food supply are making us sensitive to foods
we once tolerated, possibly by damaging the lining of the gut. Getting
to the bottom of the issue is a bit like getting to the bottom of the
Mariana Trench. Until more research is done, we won't have a good
answer on any possible link between GMOs and food sensitivities,
or any other health problems.

It's worth noting that GMOs have been banned in Europe and
Japan, and the United States doesn't require long-term studies before
genetically engineered foods can be sold.[5]

Since GMO foods aren't labeled as such in the United States, it's
not easy to avoid them. But steering clear of processed foods (a
smart move anyway) is an excellent way to start, since the majority
of processed foods in the United States contain GMOs—that's right,
the *majority*—thanks to the vast quantities of GMO soy and corn
ingredients in these products.[6] If you stick with whole foods instead
of processed foods and buy organic when you can, including organic
milk, since milk that contains RGBH, or recombinant bovine growth
hormone, is also GMO, you'll be avoiding a good amount of GMOs.
And note virtually no whole fruits or vegetables contain GMOs, with
the exception of Hawaiian papayas—so eat up!

OTHER CAUSES OF CRANKY BOWELS

When I see a patient with IBS symptoms, I generally will make sure they don't have gluten sensitivity, celiac disease, lactose intolerance or fructose intolerance. I also screen for inflammatory bowel disease (IBD) and colon cancer, as well as MTHFR mutations. (Read Gail's story earlier in this chapter.) Inflammatory bowel disease includes Crohn's disease and ulcerative colitis. These diseases are autoimmune diseases in which the body turns on itself, involving the colon and/or the small bowel and causes serious inflammation. In addition, they cause blood and mucus in the stool, pain and often weight loss. They also increase a person's risk for colon cancer.[7] As you can imagine, the work-up for all this can get quite expensive. Often I see patients who have no insurance. If you'd like to do some investigating on your own before undergoing tests, an elimination diet is a very low-cost way to rule out lactose, fructose or gluten intolerance. If an elimination diet doesn't help, you may need a colonoscopy to rule out serious problems, including IBD and colon cancer.

IBD AND COLON CANCER

IBD is an umbrella term that includes Crohn's disease and ulcerative colitis. As we explained above, people with IBD have diarrhea and cramping, as well as mucus and often blood in the stool. IBD also can cause unexplained weight loss.

Colon cancer can cause a change in bowel habits, or there may be no symptoms. If you are normally constipated and you start having frequent diarrhea, that could be reason for concern. If you normally have diarrhea, and for no apparent reason you become constipated, that's also a red flag. Some people may notice their stools are narrowing.

A colonoscopy will help to identify IBD and rule out colon cancer and will probably be performed before a diagnosis of IBS is given.

BACTERIAL OVERGROWTH

Bacterial overgrowth occurs when the number of bacteria that normally live in our gut increases significantly. Our stomach acid usually controls the number of bacteria, but now that many people are taking acid blocking drugs such as Prilosec or other acid lowering medications, such as Tagamet or Zantac, the bacteria numbers can then grow unchecked. Another cause of overgrowth is a problem with the intestine, for example decreased motility (movement) of the intestines, due to diabetes or a disease such as IBD. Poor motility allows "bad" bacteria to thrive.

The treatment is to address the underlying cause in the case of patients with motility issues or IBD. Antibiotics are also used to reduce the number of bacteria. Probiotics—supplements of "good" bacteria—help to repopulate the gut with healthy bacteria, which help keep "bad" bacteria in check. There is actually more to this story that you will read in Part II.

MTHFR MUTATIONS

We discussed the MTHFR (methylenetetrahydrofolate reductase) gene in Gail's story earlier in this chapter. This is the gene that codes for metabolism of folic acid. As I mentioned earlier, mutations in the MTHFR gene can cause the body to have problems producing serotonin, which is important to the gut as well as the brain. (Our gut is lined with cells that look like brain cells, and they secrete serotonin, which helps keep the intestinal tract running smoothly.) If you have IBS, you should be tested for a mutation of this gene. If you have one or more mutations, a supplement of L-methylfolate—a simple vitamin—could be the answer to your problems.

WHEN ALL YOUR TESTS ARE NEGATIVE

Suppose you've turned over every rock and found no cause for your digestive troubles. Some doctors would then say, "It's all in your head," and there may be some truth to that—but not in the way it sounds.

In many of the patients I see whose tests are negative, I find a past trauma at the root of their problem. When I speak to my GI colleagues, they confirm this trend.

One multicenter study of gastroenterology patients found of those with IBS, an astounding 44 percent reported a past history of sexual abuse.[8]

Another study, this one from the Mayo Clinic, confirmed non-sexual traumas also contribute to IBS. That study found IBS patients are more likely than the rest of the population to have lived through physical or mental abuse, a natural disaster, a house fire, a car accident, or other trauma.[9]

Any emotional episode can temporarily upset anyone's intestines, but what's the link between trauma and IBS? That's not clear. It could be that trauma changes signals from the brain that control nerves in the gut. Or it may sensitize the brain and the gut in a way that leads to IBS. People with IBS may also be extra-sensitive to the normal stretching of the bowel that happens with gas and with bowel movements.

For patients with IBS and a history of trauma, I prescribe eye movement desensitization and reprocessing (EMDR) therapy, a specialized type of psychotherapy. As discussed earlier, it helps patients process traumatic memories with the aid of eye movements, or tapping, or other sounds. It is extremely effective and has helped to eliminate IBS symptoms for these patients. (See Chapter 6 for more detailed information on EMDR.)

If symptoms persist or I cannot find any other reason for their IBS, I often prescribe acupuncture or hypnosis. The effectiveness of acupuncture for IBS patients has been studied and the results are inconclusive; some studies have found it helps, and others have found no effect. Many of my patients have found relief, so I regularly recommend these therapies.

The studies of hypnosis for IBS have been more positive. A review of 14 studies concluded hypnosis is quite effective for resolving the symptoms of IBS.[10]

IBS symptoms are variable and can be treated in a multitude of ways. The majority of my patients are able to resolve their symptoms through diet and alternative treatments. The key is to get to the bottom (pardon the pun) of what's going on, and then find the appropriate therapy.

4 THE BRAIN

THE STORY

Joanne was an 82 year-old-woman who had been a brilliant, successful dynamo most of her life. She lived in a major city with a demanding, fast-paced job, which she did with efficiency and enthusiasm. In her late seventies, things started to shift. She started forgetting things. It started with names and directions. Then her personality started to change. She became paranoid. She felt as if she was being watched. She started hiding things around the house. When she went out to restaurants, she tried to sneak silverware into her purse. She would forget she ate dinner and order another meal.

As time went on, Joanne became more of a recluse. Her body remained healthy as her mind started slipping away. She became very childlike. At first, she was gaining weight because she was eating multiple meals. However, she gradually forgot how to eat and swallow. She started losing weight and became very thin. Finally, she forgot how to drink water, and she died.

To the very end, there would be tiny moments of recognition that gave a fleeting glimpse of the person she used to be, and then the person she had become would be back. It was so hard for everyone around her to watch her progression. It was hard for me as well. Joanne was my mother-in-law.

Experts and Evidence

Whenever I ask patients what their biggest fear is regarding their health, the answer is fairly unanimous. They are most afraid of losing their minds. If you gave people a choice between getting cancer or Alzheimer's, the vast majority would pick cancer.

According to the Alzheimer's Association, as of 2016, more than five million Americans are living with Alzheimer's disease. Every 67 seconds, another person is developing this form of dementia. It is estimated 500,000 people die as a result of the disease every year. However, that number is falsely low. This is because this statistic is taken from death certificates, and although many a patient may have Alzheimer's disease leading to a variety of events that result in death (such as a fractured hip or a head injury or an infection), the disease is not listed as the cause of death. The immediate cause of death is what is placed on the death certificate.[1]

WHAT IS ALZHEIMER'S DISEASE?

Alzheimer's disease is a progressive disease of the brain that destroys memory and thinking skills. It generally appears in the mid-60 age group and beyond, but it can appear earlier. It is the most common cause of dementia in the elderly.

In 1906, Dr. Alois Alzheimer noticed changes in the brain tissue of a 55-year-old woman named Auguste D. who died of an unusual mental illness. At the age of 50, she was described as having memory loss, language problems and unpredictable behavior. After she died, he examined her brain and found abnormal clumps of a material we now call amyloid. There were tangled bundles of fibers as well. These are now considered the main pathologic features of the disease. Unfortunately, at the time his colleagues showed little interest in his findings. However, a fellow physician did diagnose a male patient, Josef F., with Alzheimer's disease before he died. The patient lived three years with the disease. He died at the age of 51. An autopsy was done showing the plaque without the tangles. It wasn't until 1995 when the slides from Josef F. and others were intensively reviewed that Dr. Alzheimer was credited with showing the progression of the disease in different stages. You might be wondering why others in the early 1900s did not jump on board and readily acknowledge the disease. One of the reasons may be that it was not prevalent. In 1900, the average life expectancy was 47-years-of-age. Since Alzheimer's shows up later in life, there were relatively few who had the disease.[2]

WHAT ARE THE SIGNS?

PERSONALITY CHANGE

The first thing I have noticed in my patients who have developed Alzheimer's disease is a loss of sense of humor. I remember a patient of mine from many years ago. Her name was Jan. She was a Japanese woman who had married a serviceman and moved to Oregon. Jan raised a family and was looking forward to traveling after her husband retired from his job. She was one of my favorite patients because she was so fun and bubbly. I cared for her prior to retirement, and then she left the area. Roughly ten years later, her husband brought Jan to see me. She was no longer the fun-loving, jovial person whom I remembered. Furthermore, she did not know who I was. It was alarming to say the least. She was diagnosed with advanced Alzheimer's disease; sadly, she died about a year later.

In addition to losing her sense of humor, Jan had developed paranoia and delusions. This is also common in the disease. She repeatedly called the police because she thought her husband was holding her captive. She would lock herself in the bathroom to hide and feel safe.

OTHER SIGNS OF ALZHEIMER'S:

DISORDERED THINKING

Loss of short-term memory is another early sign. Patients commonly forget appointments, words and names. They will often have sticky notes all over as memory aids.

TROUBLE WITH VISUAL AND SPATIAL IMAGES

As the disease progresses, perception may change. Patients misjudge distances and angles. Hopefully, they stop driving because they will have great difficulty and soon become dangerous behind the wheel.

Along those lines, patients may not recognize their reflection in the mirror, leading to or increasing their paranoia. They also may have trouble distinguishing colors. One of the tests we use to diagnose the disease is asking patients to draw a clock and put in a specific time. Patients with Alzheimer's typically will not be able to visualize the clock, and are unable to place the numbers and minute and hour hands in the appropriate place.

TROUBLE PLANNING AND TRACKING

One of the first things to go is the ability to keep a checkbook. That would be for someone who has always been able to do that. (Frankly, I gave up trying to balance my checkbook in the 1980s! Thankfully for me, that test doesn't count.) Following simple tasks may become difficult. As an example, using the remote for the TV or setting a microwave may become difficult to impossible. (Again, that would be for those people who actually could do it in the first place.)

CONFUSION OF THE TIME AND DATE

Disorientation regarding time and date is a common symptom of Alzheimer's. Almost everyone tends to forget what day it is when on a vacation. However, when you are in your weekly/monthly routine, forgetting is not normal. Many patients will be unclear regarding the date, time of year or time of day.

DIFFICULTY FINDING THE CORRECT WORD

We all forget names and sometimes lose words from time to time. Alzheimer's patients lose words frequently. They often have trouble maintaining and/or following a conversation. One of my patients was quite eloquent and loved to talk. I knew something was up when she rarely would converse, and when we did talk, she would get confused and agitated.

MISPLACING THINGS AND PUTTING THEM IN UNUSUAL PLACES

One of my patients would take things and put them in very odd places. And, like my mother-in-law, she developed an affinity for silverware. She would often try to take forks and spoons from restaurants and put them in her purse. At home, her husband would find silverware all over the house, under mattresses, in the freezer, and in the laundry room. She would put the house keys in the refrigerator and the remote control in the pantry. Note: it is normal to forget where you put things. Putting them in strange places is not normal.

POOR JUDGMENT

Patients with Alzheimer's may start to make poor decisions, particularly when it comes to money. They are easy prey for telemarketers and scam artists. They lose the ability to discern what is legit and what is not. One of my patients gave the majority of her money away to her college alumni association. It was very nice of her, and the college was very appreciative, but she left nothing for her children.

HOW IS ALZHEIMER'S DISEASE DIAGNOSED?

The only way to definitively diagnose Alzheimer's is at autopsy. There are many tests that can lead to the diagnosis, but as of now there is no test that can tell with 100 percent certainty that a patient has the disease. The main tests that are used are the following:

NEUROPSYCHIATRIC TESTING

When family members and patients themselves start to notice changes as we mentioned above, the first thing most doctors order is neuropsychiatric testing. Psychologists use tests to evaluate cognitive function that allows them to come to the diagnosis. These tests include problem solving, memory, attention, counting and language skills. They are able to distinguish dementia from other problems such as depression and other emotional disorders.

MEDICAL TESTS

Blood and urine tests can help rule out other causes of memory loss. Thyroid disease, vitamin deficiencies and certain infectious diseases such as syphilis can mimic this form of dementia.

BRAIN SCANS

Brain scans such as computed tomography (CT) and magnetic resonance imaging (MRI) and positron emission tomography (PET) are quite helpful. The CT and MRI scans can show other possible causes of dementia, such as stroke and infection. They can also show the loss or shrinkage of brain tissue. There is quite a bit of excitement surrounding the use of PET scans. That is because they are able to show amyloid deposits on the brain. These are suggestive but not conclusively diagnostic for Alzheimer's disease, as some people have evidence of plaques but no disease.

WHAT ARE THE TREATMENTS?

Thus far, there are medications patients can be prescribed that help to slow the progression of the disease. These include Aricept and Namenda. While there is currently no drug that reverses or stops the ravages of Alzheimer's, there are some promising new treatments being studied.[3] Let's first talk about some treatment basics.

FOOD FOR THOUGHT (LITERALLY!)

A well-balanced diet may make a difference in keeping our brains healthy. Studies have found diets rich in green leafy vegetables as well as cruciferous vegetables such as broccoli and Brussels sprouts maintain healthy brain function.

Several studies have found when people followed the Mediterranean diet, they had a lower risk of developing Alzheimer's. One study in particular found there was a 28 percent lower risk of developing the very early stage of the disease, called mild cognitive impairment. Those who maintained the diet had a 48 percent lower risk of progressing from mild cognitive impairment to full blown Alzheimer's.[4] The Mediterranean diet is one that is rich in whole foods, which include vegetables, fruits, legumes, whole grains, lean protein, olive oil and an occasional glass of red wine.

FISH OIL MAY BE ANOTHER EFFECTIVE TOOL FOR PREVENTION

Fish oil has been found to help the memory of mice bred to have Alzheimer's. The mice develop amyloid plaque on their brains. These plaques are suspected as being part of the cause of Alzheimer's in humans. Mice who were given a diet rich in omega-3 fatty acids had fewer deposits of plaque than those who were not given the fish oil.[5]

Unfortunately, the same results have not been seen in people. It has been suggested supplementation with fish oil needs to be started early, before the cognitive decline starts happening.

NEW MEDICAL THERAPIES?

One of the other possible causes of this disease is that the brain becomes resistant to insulin. In theory, a diabetes medication called Metformin should halt and possibly reverse cognitive impairment. In fact, a study done in 2008 found patients with diabetes and Alzheimer's showed cognitive improvement after being on Metformin.[6]

A study done in the aforementioned mice has found the diabetes drug Victoza (Liraglutide) was able to expedite removal of the amyloid plaque off the brains of the mice with Alzheimer's and return their normal cognitive function. This drug is injected daily and lowers blood sugar without causing hypoglycemia or low blood sugar. The drug is currently being studied in Alzheimer's patients and is showing great promise.[7]

A small study done in Canada has found Alzheimer's patients treated with intravenous immunoglobulin showed no further cognitive decline after three treatments. Researchers believe the antibodies in the immunoglobulin halted the inflammation that causes beta amyloid to be formed in the brain. Further clinical trials on this promising treatment are ongoing as well.[8]

Researchers recently reported very exciting results of a small study called the metabolic enhancement for neurodegeneration, or MEND program, conducted with nine patients who had early Alzheimer's disease and one with advanced disease. Recognizing that single or mono-therapies have been unsuccessful in reversing the disease, they decided to try a multi-pronged approach personalized for each patient.[9]

As an example, one female patient eliminated all simple carbohydrates from her diet, resulting in a 20-pound weight loss. She eliminated all gluten and processed foods from her diet increasing her intake of fruit, vegetables and wild fish. She reduced stress with yoga and meditated 20 minutes twice a day. She took melatonin (0.5 mgs) at bedtime, vitamin D (2000 IU's daily) and CoQ10 (200 mgs daily). She started flossing regularly and used an electric toothbrush. She had stopped her hormones after the WHI study results came out in 2002 showing an increased risk for breast cancer on hormones. The MEND program doctors had her resume taking her hormone replacement therapy. She fasted at least 12 hours between dinner and breakfast, and she exercised at least 30 minutes four to five days a week. It has been two-and-a-half years, and her symptoms have reversed and she remains asymptomatic.

Others who had high cholesterol were treated to optimize their levels with diet and medication. Those who needed vitamin B12 were supplemented and others were given minerals such as copper and zinc.

Although the changes were difficult for patients to follow, the results kept them in the program, and nine out of ten have maintained their improvements. Larger trials will be forthcoming.

PARKINSON'S DISEASE

Another disease that strikes fear into people's hearts and has no cure is Parkinson's, which is a degenerative disorder of the nervous system. It is a condition which is chronic and progressive.

THE STORY

Theresa is a 65-year-old woman who had always been active. She noticed she was developing a tremor and her balance was off. She would feel as if she were falling forward when she walked. Sometimes she would just freeze and not be able to keep going. Her family noticed she no longer smiled, and her voice was a bit shaky as well. She complained of pain and stiffness in her arms. She went to her doctor, who suspected she had Parkinson's disease, and the neurologist she was referred to confirmed the diagnosis. She was treated with medications and was able to regain her movements. Ultimately, she was given a revolutionary device, which acts as a pacemaker for the brain. This has transformed her life. More on this later.

Experts and Evidence

WHAT ARE THE SYMPTOMS?

There are four main symptoms of Parkinson's disease:

TREMOR

The classic tremor in Parkinson's disease is a rhythmic back-and-forth motion that involves the thumb and forefinger and is described as pill rolling. It is most apparent at rest and disappears during sleep and improves with intentional movement.

RIGIDITY

Rigidity or a resistance to movement is another common symptom. The muscles are tense and contracted so they cause stiffness and pain.

It becomes most obvious as someone tries to move a patient's arm. It becomes rigid and resists movement and this results in a cogwheel motion.

BRADYKINESIA

Defined as an abnormal slowness of movement, the patient affected cannot perform routine movements quickly. The facial expression will also stiffen.

LOSS OF BALANCE

Parkinson's will cause patients to be unstable. They will often fall over whether standing or sitting, but Parkinson's symptoms often start on one side of the body. As the disease progresses, it affects both sides. People will start to walk with a gait that causes them to lean forward and take hurried steps. They may have trouble initiating movement and may stop suddenly as they walk and then they freeze.

OTHER SYMPTOMS

People have difficulty walking, talking and completing simple tasks. The disease eventually causes patients to become wheelchair bound or even completely bedridden. They often develop dementia. Swallowing becomes difficult and they can develop aspiration pneumonia and chronic bronchitis. Forty-four percent of patients die as a result of complications from pneumonia and bronchitis.[10]

Speech is affected in half of the patients, causing them to speak softly and in monotone. Other accompanying symptoms include: urinary difficulty, oily skin and hair, sleeping difficulties, memory problems and trouble maintaining blood pressure while standing. Fatigue and loss of energy are also quite common along with emotional changes. It is a life-changing, terribly burdensome disease.

WHO GETS IT?

It is estimated that 50,000 Americans are diagnosed with Parkinson's each year. It affects 50 percent more men than women.

The usual age of onset is around 60 years. Those with one or more close relatives with the disease are at higher risk. Scientists have identified several genetic mutations associated with Parkinson's disease.

WHAT CAUSES IT?

Parkinson's disease occurs when nerve cells in the brain die or become damaged. The main part of the brain affected is the substantia nigra. The cells in this area produce dopamine. This is a chemical messenger responsible for transmitting signals between the substantia nigra and the corpus striatum, also known as the relay station of the brain, that produces smooth movements. Loss of dopamine causes abnormal firing of these signals. Studies have found Parkinson's patients have lost 60 to 80 percent or more of their dopamine-producing cells by the time symptoms appear.[11]

Parkinson's is a disease of the entire body. It is believed the disease actually starts in the peripheral nervous system in an area such as the intestine, where symptoms can be present in the form of constipation for years before it is diagnosed.

TOXINS

There are certain toxins linked to Parkinson's disease. They may cause the disease by altering genes with mutations that look similar to those linked to hereditary Parkinson's disease.

Metal manganese and a drug known as MPTP (1-methyl-4-phenyl-1,2,3,6-tetrahydropyridine), an industrial chemical and a contaminant of illicit narcotics, have both been found to cause Parkinson's disease.[12]

DRUGS

Certain drugs that are prescribed for patients with psychiatric problems such as chlorpromazine and haloperidol can cause a reversible form of Parkinson's. Drugs, such as one used for stomach problems, metoclopramide, and a seizure medication known as valproate can also cause a reversible form of the disease.[13]

OTHER CAUSES

Damage as a result of multiple strokes can cause a type of Parkinson's disease. Similarly, frequent head injury, such as that seen in boxers like Muhammad Ali, can also cause the disease. A viral infection may be another potential cause.

THE STORY

I would like to share my grandmother's story to give some thoughts and perspective. She was born in 1900, but she was definitely not a typical Victorian of the "weaker sex." My grandmother was a self-sufficient businesswoman. She prided herself on being independent. She traveled all over the world.

Later in her life, at age 75, she developed Parkinson's. There is some evidence as to why. As a child, she had been afflicted by the Spanish flu epidemic in 1918. At that time, there was a severe outbreak of the flu that killed millions worldwide, including at least 675,000 Americans.[14] She talked about that time in history when so many people she knew lost their lives; it was a terribly frightening time for those who had to live through it. Those who did felt lucky to have survived. Unfortunately, these survivors found themselves at higher risk of developing Parkinson's disease directly following the exposure and as well later in life, suggesting there is an infectious component to developing the disease.[15] I believe my grandmother was one of those afflicted. It was a sorrow and an ordeal that affected our whole family.

TREATMENTS

There is currently no cure for Parkinson's disease. Treatment is aimed at reducing symptoms. This is done by boosting dopamine levels or keeping it from being broken down and picked up by receptors so more is available to the brain or by using drugs that mimic dopamine. There are a variety of medications such as L–Dopa that can help. There is also a type of brain surgery that has been effective. A pacemaker is placed in the globus pallidus, which is in the basal ganglia. This stimulation improves Parkinson's symptoms. It is a fairly extreme treatment and is used for those who have failed medications.[16]

THE IMPORTANCE OF EXERCISE

Staying flexible and mobile is essential. It is important for the body but also for the soul. In Part IV, we describe a very effective form of exercise that actually allows the body to bypass the damaged part of the brain. Stay tuned. Or, if you can't help yourself, skip ahead and check it out now.

TRAUMATIC BRAIN INJURY (TBI)

THE STORY

John, a 19-year-old competitive dancer, was returning from a dance competition and had car trouble. He pulled his car over to the side of the road to wait for a tow truck. As he was waiting, he took a bite of a sandwich he had packed, and at the same time was hit by a guy driving and texting at 80 miles per hour. Not only was his seat belt sheared off, the impact caused him to aspirate his sandwich and block his trachea. He had a severe cervical spine injury and was comatose for over a week.

When he came to, he had difficulty walking, talking and thinking clearly. No one expected him to make a full recovery. He underwent intensive rehabilitation, and with the help of a certain special activity (which we will discuss in detail soon), he is completely back and better than ever.

Experts and Evidence

Traumatic brain injury, also known as TBI, is a problem that has increased in the modern era. It is an acquired brain injury.

Best described by the National Institutes of Health, a TBI occurs when physical, external forces impact the brain either from a penetrating object or a bump, blow, or jolt to the head. Not all blows or jolts to the head result in a TBI. For the ones that do, TBI can range from mild (a brief change in mental status or consciousness) to severe (an extended period of unconsciousness or amnesia after the injury).

TBI affects between 2.5 and 6.5 million Americans. Survivors are often left with significant cognitive, behavioral and communicative disabilities.

WHAT ARE THE CAUSES?

According to data from the Centers for Disease Control and Prevention (CDC) and the National Institutes of Health, falls are the most common cause of TBI and occur most frequently among the youngest and oldest age groups. From 2006 to 2010 alone, falls caused more than half (55 percent) of TBI among children aged 14 and younger. Among Americans age 65 and older, **falls accounted for more than two-thirds (81 percent) of all reported TBI.**

The second and third most common causes of TBI are unintentional blunt trauma (accidents that involved being struck by or against an object), followed closely by motor vehicle accidents. Blunt trauma is especially common in children younger than 15 years old, causing nearly a quarter of all TBI. Assaults account for an additional 10 percent of TBI, and include abuse-related TBI, such as head injuries that result from shaken baby syndrome.

Half of TBI incidents in adults involve alcohol. The severity of the outcome is related to the cause. Ninety-one percent of TBI due to firearms result in death, whereas only 11 percent of falls result in death.

TYPES OF TBI

There are many different types of brain injuries that vary depending on the severity and type of injury. There are two broad types of head injuries: penetrating and non-penetrating.

Penetrating TBI (also known as *open* TBI) occurs when the skull is pierced by an object (for example, a bullet, shrapnel, bone fragment, or by a weapon such as hammer, knife, or baseball bat). With this injury, the object enters the brain tissue.

Non-penetrating TBI (also known as *closed head injury* or *blunt* TBI) is caused by an external force that produces movement of the brain within the skull. Causes include falls, motor vehicle crashes, sports injuries, or being struck by an object. Blast injury due to explosions is a focus of intense study, but how it causes brain injury is not fully known.

One of the most common types of injury is concussion *from a non-penetrating injury.* It is a type of mild TBI that may be considered a temporary injury to the brain but could take minutes to several months to heal. Concussion can be caused by a number of things, including a bump, a blow or a jolt to the head, a sports injury or fall, a motor vehicle accident, a weapons blast, or a rapid acceleration or deceleration of the brain within the skull (such as the person having been violently shaken). Beyond concussion, the injuries can increase in severity depending on the cause ranging from blood clots, severe bruising and bleeding to skull fractures.[17]

COMPLICATIONS

Depending on the severity of the injury, complications can occur. Seizures, infection, pain and injuries of the nerves to the face are among them. Twenty-five percent of those with brain contusions or hematomas, and 50 percent of patients with penetrating head trauma develop seizures immediately. Headache is the most common symptom of TBI. Even those with mild injury can suffer post-concussion syndrome. The symptoms include: headache, dizziness, vertigo, memory problems, trouble concentrating, sleeping problems, restlessness, irritability, apathy, depression and anxiety. Many patients may have trouble speaking and writing, and they may have visual perception problems.

These types of head injuries also increase the risk for Parkinson's disease, Alzheimer's disease and post-traumatic dementia.[18]

WHAT CAN BE DONE?

Physical rehabilitation is essential. In addition, speech therapy and occupational therapy and even visual therapy may be required.

PREVENTION

The best solution to the problem of TBI is to avoid it in the first place. The important thing is to wear a seatbelt when riding in a car and wear a helmet riding a bicycle or a motorcycle. We live in Oregon, and it's amazing how many bicyclists around here choose *not* to wear a helmet. Of course we are referring to most *adult* bike riders as opposed to the kids, whom we never see riding without their helmets. We surmise when people get older, they start thinking they've grown immune to head injury, and they believe their heads are somehow harder and have become impact-resistant. To say these people are fooling themselves is an understatement. Be sure to also keep those helmets on when playing football, baseball, rollerblading or riding a skateboard. And keep them on for winter sports too: snowboarding, skiing, ice skating and hockey.

Finally, keep all guns locked away along with the bullets. GSI (gunshot injuries also known as GSW or gunshot wounds) make for the worst TBI of all.

"Surviving is important. Thriving is elegant."

—MAYA ANGELOU

Part II
WHAT'S NEW?

INTRODUCTION

As you can observe from all the studies and information being discussed on television, radio and the Internet, there is almost a continuous flow of new information regarding health and wellness. It is very hard for most of us to sift through it all to figure out what is important and what is not. In Part II, we are going to help you with that. There are some new things available now and some others coming not too far down the road. You will like learning about them, and many may be essential for your personal health. This is going to be fun!

5 LONGEVITY

UNFORTUNATELY, WE STILL don't know why our bodies age. There are many theories and scientists are very busy trying to figure out the answer. One theory is that our genes determine how long we live. Another theory is our DNA becomes damaged over time; it can't recover and this ultimately leads to our demise.

Telomeres act as protective caps on the end of our chromosomes, which make up our DNA and get shorter as we age. Stem cells make an enzyme called *telomerase* to replenish the telomeres, but most telomeres shrink with every division over time, so the cells will start to fade or die. We know telomere damage effects aging from studies done on mice. Those with short telomeres live shorter lives. In humans, mutated telomerase is associated with an increased risk of cancer. The telomeres are at increased risk of damage from outside stress, which might explain the differences in how individuals age.[1]

There is another theory that mitochondria are behind the aging process. Mitochondria are the power stations of our cells. They have their own pool of DNA. The DNA in mitochondria get more mutations than the DNA elsewhere. When the mitochondria make energy, they create what we call oxidative stress. This can damage DNA. That is why those who eat less may live longer. Less food leads to less oxidative stress.[2]

An experiment done in Sweden found this theory was correct when it came to mice. When they accelerated the mitochondrial mutations in a set of mice, the animals lived about one year as opposed to two to three years in mice left to age normally.[3]

There is yet another very interesting theory about aging that deals with the cells themselves. Scientists have found the aging process causes regulators to be released that circulate in the blood. One of them is called growth differentiation factor 11, or GDF11. This controls gene expression in patterns by lining up organs in order in the body from front to back. The level of GDF-11 decreases with age. A group of Harvard Medical School researchers surgically joined young and old mice. They found the young blood restored some of the lost function of the heart, brains and skeletal muscles of the older mice, and using GDF11 alone actually gave the same result.[4] The next question is, would treating humans with GDF11 do the same thing? Time and research will tell. In the meantime, there are many things we can do.

Genetics is responsible for about 25 percent of how we age. The rest has to do with lifestyle choices and environmental exposures. What is interesting is that organs in the same person age at different rates based on the above factors.[5]

Here are some reminders you have likely already heard and hopefully you've already heeded. To preserve the skin, avoid the sun or use hats and sunscreen. To preserve lung and cardiac function, do not start smoking. If you smoke, quit. Exercise on a regular basis and eat a heart-healthy diet (The Mediterranean diet discussed in Chapter 7). For a healthy gut, eat a healthy diet and do your regular screenings for colon cancer starting at age 50 or sooner, depending on your family history. Having a healthy gut affects the rest of your body, as you will see later on in this section of the book. For a healthy brain, exercise, eat well and read and follow Part IV.

GOOD NEWS

Now to the fun part of the longevity story. The epidemiologic and psychological pieces explaining why people live long and thrive are huge. There are several landmark studies.

Since 1976, The National Institutes of Health have been studying the Okinawans, where living to 100 is commonplace. What they have found is the following:[6]

- Elderly Okinawans exercise physically and mentally.
- They eat a diet low in salt and high in fruits and vegetables.
- They eat between 60 to 120 grams of soy a day. Theirs is *not* genetically modified. Soy is high in flavonoids. These are compounds found in plant pigments. They are powerful antioxidants and anti-inflammatories.
- They do not overeat. They stop before they become full. They usually eat around 1800 calories a day.
- Their diet is high in vitamin E, which may be why they have less dementia.[7]
- Elderly Okinawans are highly regarded and feel they are a vital part of their communities.

This study confirms the need for a healthy diet, stress release and the importance of a supportive community for long life.

What about those who live long lives here in the United States? In 1921, Louis Terman, a psychologist at Stanford University, launched a study of more than 1500 bright children who were about ten years old. They followed these children throughout their lives and studied family histories, relationships, hobbies, pets, job and educational success and many other factors. The original plan was to study them for six months. It continues today.[8] Here are some of the key findings:

- Marriage is important for men's health, but not for women. Men who stayed in long-term marriages were more likely to make it past 70. Less than a third of divorced men made it beyond 70. Men who never married lived longer than divorced men, but not as long as married men.

- Being divorced was much less harmful to women's health. It did not affect life expectancy.
- Those who were involved and committed to their jobs lived longer than those who were not. Productivity is important.
- Those who began first grade before age six were at higher risk for early mortality. Kids need to play.
- Playing with pets is not associated with a longer life.
- Combat veterans are at risk for early mortality. It is due to unhealthy patterns rather than the trauma itself. Those who were able to find meaning in the experience were more likely to find a healthy way to live.

And . . .

- There is yet more information from another landmark longevity study still ongoing. It is the Grant Study of Harvard Alumni. The research was started in 1938. It examined 268 members of Harvard classes between 1939 and 1944. Two of the distinguished members of the study were John F. Kennedy and famed newspaper editor Ben Bradlee. (As an interesting aside, Leonard Bernstein and Norman Mailer were rejected.) The research initially involved rigorous physical exams, and follow-ups over years. In 1966, the study started to take a look at the subjects from a psychological as well as a physical perspective.[9]

The study also included 456 men from inner-city Boston between 1940 and 1945 that were studied as controls for juvenile delinquency. They were added to the study in the 1970s. Many of the participants have lived into their 80s and 90s and Harvard is now doing the Second Generation Study, learning about the children of the original participants.

The subjects answer extensive questionnaires every two years. They also do in-depth interviews and have recently submitted to DNA blood tests and neuroimaging. Now, their wives have been asked to engage in the interview process.

There are so many things that have been learned from this study that there have been three books written, and there are more on the way. Some of the things that have been revealed:

- Having a tough childhood has a significant impact on early adulthood.
- The effects of a difficult childhood fade over time.
- Those who are self-starters and get jobs as kids live longer than those who do not.
- College is important for determining lifetime success (more than money or social status).
- One's situation at age 50 has more to do with health and happiness at 70 than what happened earlier in life.
- The ability to play in childhood is a better indicator of late-life happiness than income.
- A stable marriage is correlated to late-life happiness.
- Alcohol was a major factor in 57 percent of the divorces in the Grant Study.
- Although genetics plays a role, lifestyle choices have a huge impact on longevity and happiness.

This study confirms the value of adopting a healthy lifestyle for wellbeing as well as for physical health. It's also encouraging to know one can get over a difficult childhood and still happily thrive after 50; the resilience of the human spirit—and the human body—has been proven once again![10]

6 DEPRESSION

ONE OF THOSE things that can affect longevity in a big way is depression. A recent VA evaluation of over five million veterans studied in the year 2007 found depression was a major cause of early mortality. In this group, depression was associated with early death and a loss of productive life—more than all 13 causes of death that were examined. These included strokes, accidents, diabetes, heart disease, homicide, flu and pneumonia, liver disease, cancer, kidney disease, lung disease, infection and suicide.[1]

> **THE STORY**
>
> Depression always loomed in Thalia's life. At 60 years old and looking back, she could not remember a time when she was happy. She grew up an only child with a mother who was emotionally absent and who suffered from bipolar disorder. Her mother's moods were unpredictable, and Thalia never felt safe. As she grew older, her depression worsened. Medications, including antidepressants, didn't help.

She was hospitalized multiple times and was treated with electroshock therapy. Still her depression persisted.

She came to see me as a last-ditch effort to find a treatment that would work. First, I normalized her thyroid levels with thyroid medication. I also did a genetic test that showed that her ability to metabolize folic acid, a B vitamin, was impaired.

I gave Thalia a prescription for 15 milligrams of L-methylfolate along with a small amount of Prozac. In addition, she went for EMDR. This helped her to resolve her issues with her mother.

About a month later, I received a phone call from Thalia. She told me for the first time in her life she was happy! She felt like it was nothing short of a miracle. It was a combination of good medicine, psychology and proper supplementation.

Experts and Evidence

Some days it feels like we're in the midst of a major depression epidemic. So many of the patients I see, especially the women, are struggling to find life a happy place, to remember what it's like to wake up looking forward to something. Here are the numbers: Almost one out of ten adults has depression at any given time. Of those, 4.1 percent have major (clinical) depression, the most serious form. But the rates among women are significantly higher. In fact, women are 70 percent more likely to suffer from depression than men.[2]

It's no surprise, then, that antidepressants are the most commonly prescribed drugs for adults ages 18 to 44, or that a whopping 11 percent of all Americans over age 12 are on one of these medications.[3] What is very surprising is how well these drugs work—or rather, *don't* work: Despite their enormous popularity, they aren't all that helpful. Less than half of people who take an antidepressant see their depression disappear. And many people stop taking the drugs due to side effects such as weight gain and loss of libido.[4]

Life with depression is both unhappy and physically damaging. It unleashes a cascade of biological and behavioral effects that can make just about every aspect of your health worse. Fortunately, the answer to "Do I have to feel like this forever?" is an emphatic "NO." Read on to discover therapies that work for my patients and can be used alone or in conjunction with antidepressants.

WHAT IF YOU NEED MEDICATION?

Some people need medication. If that is the case, it is often hard to figure out which drug to choose. I had always wondered how nice it would be if there was a road map or manual. Now, I have found the solution. There is a genetic test that gives me a framework of medications to work with. It helps me to see which medications a patient metabolizes normally and which ones they do not. This test actually extends to antipsychotics, pain medications and even medicine for ADD and ADHD. I will explain.

We are all born with a unique makeup of genes that code our DNA. They code for everything, our sex, our appearance and how our body works. Genes also code for the enzymes, the things that break down drugs in our liver. Many medications are metabolized there. There is an entire system of enzymes called Cytochrome P450 that do the work. The gene test that I do with a simple cheek swab, called GeneSight, determines the unique way the major enzymes of the liver metabolize the drugs that go through this system. It looks at the individual enzyme activity but also multiple enzymes' activity that may all impact how we metabolize a certain drug.

This test has been literally a lifesaver for many. There is no way to look at someone and tell if a drug is going to be harmful to them. By looking at how things are metabolized, I have a much better idea. The test will tell me if someone is a normal metabolizer, a slow or a rapid or an ultra-rapid metabolizer. If they are normal, there is a lower risk of an adverse reaction. If they are a slow metabolizer, they may experience side effects at the usual dose of a medication, and it may not work very well. If they are a rapid or an ultra-rapid metabolizer, the drug may not build up a blood level of the medication so it can work at the usual dosage; thus more may be needed.

With a very simple printout, I can see if a drug has a high likelihood of causing a significant reaction. If so, it would be in the red zone. If it is questionable, it is in the yellow zone, and if it doesn't have a known gene-drug interaction, it is in the green zone.

In full disclosure, I have been so impressed with the results of the test I speak for the company to educate other physicians about it. I do get paid an honorarium, but I would do it regardless because this test has revolutionized my practice.

It is amazing how many people were getting sick from the medications that were supposed to be helping them to get better. I had one patient who was on so many medications she wasn't metabolizing that when I stopped them all, she felt normal again. That is what was making her sick. I now do the test before I start a patient on any antidepressant or pain medication.

I highly recommend you have this test done if you are on antidepressants or contemplating going on them. If you have children who need medication for depression, pain or ADD/ADHD, this test should be done. Ritalin is the usual starting medication, but studies have found 30 percent of those started on it will have an adverse reaction.[5] It is easy to do. Think about it. You can find out more at https://genesight.com/.

WHAT IF YOU DON'T NEED MEDICATION?

The L-methylfolate Miracle

Thalia's depression, like many people's, was rooted in part in genetics. In her case, she had two mutations on a very important gene. The gene, called methylenetetrahydrofolate reductase, or MTHFR, mentioned earlier in Chapter 3, codes for an enzyme without which it's hard to feel good. That's because without it, you won't have enough of the feel-good hormone serotonin.

The enzyme in question turns folic acid, also known as vitamin B9, into L-methylfolate, an active form of the vitamin. L-methylfolate has a lot of important functions. The one that affects mood is helping the body produce the brain chemicals serotonin, norepinephrine and dopamine (collectively known as neurotransmitters), which play a critical role in mood regulation.

In short, defects in the MTHFR gene mean too little serotonin—and not enough happiness. And it turns out these defects are incredibly common. Scientists have reported finding as many as 40 different mutations on MTHFR! And in the United States, up to 60 percent of us have a mutation in one copy of the gene (remember, you have two copies of every gene, one from each parent), and up to 25 percent of people have at least one mutation on both copies. Having one mutation reduces your ability to convert folic acid by 34 percent. Having two mutations reduces it by 71 percent! [6]

The treatment is simple: a regular daily dose of L-methylfolate. Yes, a vitamin—you don't even need a prescription! Taken in the right amounts (7.5 to 15 milligrams per day), it can improve mild depression relatively quickly. In a study of elderly depressed patients, the response rate at six weeks was an amazing 81 percent. Results are often seen in just two weeks.[7]

If you're taking an antidepressant and aren't getting enough relief, taking L-methylfolate might help. A recent study of people with major depression found adding 15 milligrams of the supplement to an antidepressant regimen doubled the improvement in depression symptoms over a period of 30 days.[8]

L-methylfolate is well tolerated, causing no more side effects than a placebo.[9] And it doesn't interact with other medications. The results I've seen are impressive. When I treat people who have MTHFR mutations—even people who aren't depressed—with L-methylfolate, their mood improves. They may find they feel happier and are better able to handle daily stress, and often, they sleep better. Related problems such as irritable bowel syndrome will often get better as well.

If you are depressed, whether or not you take an antidepressant, ask your doctor to test you for a MTHFR defect. All it takes is a blood sample or cheek swab. If your serotonin levels are genetically low, why not find out if a simple vitamin supplement can boost them? The test is Medicare approved and is no longer considered experimental.

Most insurance companies cover the MTHFR blood test, and a few will even cover the cheek swab.

EMDR: HELP FOR COPING WITH PAST TRAUMA

THE STORY

Gail is a 60-year-old woman who had raised her grandson on her own. They were very close. As a boy, he saved his money and bought her a gold necklace for her birthday. When he turned 18, she bought him a pickup-truck as a gift. One night not long after, he rolled the truck, hit a tree and was killed. Gail was devastated. I saw her two years after the event. She still could not stop crying. I suggested EMDR therapy. She fought me tooth and nail, but recognized the pain was unbearable, so she finally went.

It took four sessions. After her last session, she came to see me and proclaimed the therapy hadn't worked. I pointed out to her she was no longer crying and she was strong in her defiance. She realized she did indeed feel stronger.

The therapist had suggested at her fourth session she take off the necklace her grandson had given her. She told me that was never going to happen. Six months later, she came for a visit. The necklace was off. She was happy and agreed EMDR was the best thing she had ever done. She was able to remember her grandson with love and focus on her happy memories of him.

Experts and Evidence

Depression is complicated. Genes, lifestyle choices and past experiences, even diet and exercise all can affect our moods. I have found psychotherapy can be very helpful for some patients, along with other modalities.

Often I find people who are depressed are suffering from symptoms of post-traumatic stress disorder (PTSD). They have had a trauma in their life that influences how they see the world. Some have been molested and abused, some have witnessed horrible events, and some have experienced things that would boggle anyone's mind. For that reason, as I did with Gail in the story above, I often recommend EMDR therapy.

EMDR, eye movement desensitization reprocessing, is an established therapy psychologists use to help resolve PTSD. It's based on the theory that strong emotions during a traumatic event can interrupt the normal information processing that happens when a memory is formed. Basically, in the moment of trauma, the sympathetic nervous system becomes overwhelmed. As a result, the memory is never fully processed by the brain, and the extremely unpleasant emotions of the moment, and even the physical sensations, are stored along with the memory. The goal of EMDR is to help the patient fully process the memory so it's stored appropriately in the brain—without the over-the-top or inappropriate emotions and physical responses the memory currently evokes. It is quite remarkable and effective for people who've experienced major traumas and may also help people who have been through less dramatic but still upsetting experiences.

EMDR is a complex process, but it boils down to this: the patient is asked to summon a mental image of the distressing event. As she focuses on that mental image, she follows with her eyes the therapist's fingers, which move side to side across her field of vision, usually for about 30 seconds at a time. EMDR practitioners explain these eye movements disrupt working (short-term) memory and create a state similar to lucid dreaming. Eventually, after the process is repeated a number of times, the patient should feel no distress when conjuring the memory.

At that point, the therapist repeats the eye movement exercises while this time the patient thinks of a more positive memory or belief.[10]

Essentially, EMDR takes the "fear charge" from memories, says Jan Baker, PhD, the clinical psychologist I refer patients to. "After releasing the fear charge, the person feels detached from any strong negative emotions associated with that experience," says Baker, who specializes in EMDR. She notes therapies like EMDR can help when talk therapy can't. " The 'shock imprint' of the experience is so deep in the nervous system verbal therapy just won't do it." In her practice, it usually takes three or four sessions to "dissolve" the memory circuit associated with the traumatic event. "It literally changes people's lives."

More than a dozen good-quality studies have shown EMDR to be helpful, and it's been recognized as an effective treatment by organizations such as the American Psychiatric Association as well as the Department of Defense.[11]

If you want to try EMDR, ask your doctor for a referral, or call the EMDR institute or go to their website at www.EMDR.com. Dr. Baker recommends you find someone in your area who has had two levels of certification and has a significant number of years of experience with the therapy.

OTHER NATURAL THERAPIES

There are many other supplements patients may try for depression since they are over the counter. It is important to know about them before you try them. I'll touch on two of the most popular ones here.

St. John's Wort has been shown in the majority of studies to help with mild to moderate depression. A potential negative of taking this herb is it interacts with a large number of medications. It shouldn't be taken with antidepressants. Another significant problem is the amount of the most important ingredient, hypercin, can vary widely from one brand to the next, so it's very hard to know when or if you're getting a therapeutic dose.

The second supplement, SAMe, is popular for depression, and some studies show it does work. There's also evidence it can boost the effectiveness of antidepressants. I use it for joint health more than mental health. A main reason I don't recommend it often is it gets awfully expensive—well over $100 a month—if you take the dosages that help with depression.[12]

EXERCISE AS AN ANTIDEPRESSANT

Regular exercise makes us feel good physically. It also can help with depression. In a landmark study done in 1999, researchers took 156 men and women and divided them into three groups. One group followed an aerobic exercise program, another took the antidepressant Zoloft and a third group did both. At the end of 16 weeks, they all had improved. In fact, 60 to 70 percent of people across all the groups were no longer considered to have major depression. This means the exercise worked as well as the antidepressant (and with far fewer side effects)! After six months, the researchers checked in with the patients again and found those in the exercise-only group were less likely to have relapsed than those who took medication and didn't exercise.[13]

What kind of exercise should you do? The kind you're most likely to keep doing! Find something you like and make it part of your life. It could be bicycling, running, hiking or dancing. The key is to get moving and *keep* moving. The more you exercise, the better you'll feel. More on this in Part IV.

IS YOUR DIET MAKING YOU DEPRESSED?

Depression can be due in part to genetics, but the truth is lifestyle choices, including diet, can play a major role. Remember the documentary *Supersize Me?* The director and star, Morgan Spurlock, was a fit, happy guy who was feeling great. Then he decided to eat McDonalds three times a day for a month and document the effects. In the course of that month, he gained 24.5 pounds, his body mass index increased 13 percent, and he was aching all over. He also became moody and depressed.

If that could happen to someone in the course of one month of eating fast food, think about the impact over years—or a lifetime. And you don't have to have supersized yourself to feel the effects of a poor diet, especially if that diet is lacking the following nutrients linked to mood:

THE B-HAPPY VITAMINS

One problem with a McDonald's-type diet is a lack of folate. Folate, also known as folic acid or vitamin B9, found in green leafy vegetables, nuts, and fruits, is important for the production of brain chemicals such as serotonin, dopamine and norepinephrine. In one study, a third of depressed adults were found to have low levels of folic acid. Another study found when depressed patients on Prozac were given a folic acid supplement, their depression improved significantly more than patients who didn't take the supplement.[14]

The solution for most people is simple: Eat more fruits and leafy greens. If you're eating plenty of vegetables, you probably don't need a supplement. If you do need one, ask your doctor about taking a B-complex supplement which will provide folic acid and other B vitamins. One good product is Super B-Complex by Nature Made. Of course, if a genetic test shows you have an MTHFR mutation (discussed earlier in this chapter), you'll need supplements of L-methylfolate, the active form of folic acid.

Vitamin B12 is another "B happy" vitamin. A hamburger diet may provide plenty of B12, since red meat is a good source, but too much red meat could eventually kill you.[15] Other better-for-you animal products that contain B12 include chicken, fish, seafood, and eggs. If you take a proton-pump inhibitor such as Prilosec (to reduce stomach acid) or birth control pills, you may be prone to B12 deficiency. In addition, many people start to have trouble absorbing B12 from food as they age.

If a blood test shows your levels are low and you suspect one of your medications is to blame, a B-complex supplement might solve the problem. If you're older, consider taking B12 strips that melt under your tongue, available at health-food stores. With these strips, absorption in the stomach isn't an issue. The other alternative is B12 shots. (A spray is also available, but it's ridiculously expensive.) The daily-recommended intake of B12 for adults is 2.4 micrograms, and it's a good idea to have your proper amount for many reasons.

Having adequate B12 levels is important for mood and probably for the treatment of depression as well. A study of 115 people in Finland who were being treated for depression found people with higher levels of B12 responded better to treatment with an antidepressant over a six-month period compared to those with lower levels.[16]

One last B vitamin, vitamin B6, or pyridoxine, is also important for the formation of serotonin. If you take birth control pills, your levels of B6 may be low. I tell all my patients on oral contraceptives to take a vitamin B supplement. If you're not on the pill and you are a healthy eater with a diet that includes green leafy vegetables, bananas, nuts and seeds, beans and fish (such as tuna and salmon), then you probably do not need a supplement. A survey in the United States found teenagers and young adults (between ages 21 and 44) are most likely to be deficient.[17]

The RDA for vitamin B6 is 1.3 milligrams for adults 19 to 50, 1.7 milligrams for men 51 and older, 1.5 milligrams for women 51 and older, 1.9 milligrams for pregnant women, and 2 milligrams for breastfeeding women.[18]

D IS FOR DEPRESSION

A recent study found vitamin D helped reverse moderate to severe depression in women with a D deficiency.[19] Although the study was small, the results were significant. Over a 12-week period, when women's vitamin D levels were increased from a range of 8.9 to 14.5 nanograms per milliliter (ng/ml) to between 32 and 38 ng/ml, their depression test scores markedly improved. A larger study would be welcomed, but there are already enough good reasons to maintain a healthy vitamin D level for general health.

There is no one-size-fits-all recommendation for vitamin D supplements. Some are better at making and storing vitamin D than others. Some of us live in places that get more sunlight than others, or spend more time outdoors than others. (Incidentally, you can't get vitamin D through glass since UVB rays that carry it do not penetrate glass). And if you cover all of your exposed skin with sunscreen, it doesn't matter how sunny it is, you'll have a hard time making vitamin D at all. But taking too much D is dangerous. Unlike water-soluble vitamins, which are excreted if you take too much, D is stored in the liver. The bottom line: Ask your doctor to test your blood levels of D before you start supplementing.

C YOURSELF HAPPIER

Low levels of vitamin C have been associated with depression. When researchers compared the vitamin C levels of depressed women who attempted suicide to those of women who were not depressed, their levels were significantly lower.[20] More evidence: A recent study at McGill University found people hospitalized with an acute illness or medical problem who were given vitamin C twice daily showed a 34 percent improvement in their mood scores. Seventy-four percent of the patients were vitamin C deficient at the outset.[21]

It's not hard to maintain adequate vitamin C levels; just eat plenty of colorful fruits (especially citrus fruits, berries and melons) and vegetables (especially broccoli, bell peppers and dark, leafy greens). Notice we said *fruits* and not *fruit juice*, which is loaded with sugar.

FISH OIL: NOT FISHY AT ALL

Depression has been linked to inflammation in the body, both as a cause and a result. Omega-3 fatty acids, found in fatty fish, are highly anti-inflammatory. They're also highly concentrated in the brain and are thought to be essential for healthy brain function. It's little wonder, then, that countries with higher fish consumption have less depression and bipolar disorder (a severe form of depression). Plenty of studies link eating fish or taking fish oil supplements with a lowered risk of depression. For example:

- In northern Finland, a study of more than 5,000 people found women who ate fish regularly were 2.5 times less likely to become depressed compared to those who rarely ate fish.[22]
- One study gave patients with bipolar disorder ten grams (a huge amount) of fish oil a day or placebo.

The results showed 64 percent of the patients improved on fish oil compared with just 19 percent of those given placebo.[23]

- A study in Belgium looking at fish oil levels found levels were low in patients with depression. Giving patients fish oil helped to improve their mood.[24]

Fish oil improves blood flow to the brain. It also decreases the amount of arachidonic acid, a type of unhealthy fatty acid, in the brain. Arachidonic acid is a marker for silent inflammation, and there's more of it in the cerebrospinal fluid (the fluid that bathes the brain) of depressed patients.

So how can you get enough fish oil? It's always my first choice to get nutrients from food. Aim for two 3-ounce servings of fatty cold-water fish, such as salmon, halibut or herring, a week. Large fish such as tilefish, mackerel, shark and swordfish contain higher levels of mercury and toxins and should be eaten in moderation. Catfish and tilapia contain higher levels of unhealthy fatty acids. Farm raised fish may contain pesticides and antibiotics, so I recommend wild fish.

Most of us have a hard time finding fresh wild fish year round, and it becomes difficult to eat fish twice weekly. In addition, eating ten grams of fish oil daily to treat bipolar disorder can be downright impossible. Fortunately, the majority of fish oil supplements in the United States are mercury free. They will say it right on the label. Good-quality fish oil will contain adequate amounts of docosahexaenoic acid, or DHA (at least 600 milligrams) and eicosapentaenoic acid, or EPA (at least 400 milligrams). These are the fatty acids that are good for you. When you buy fish oil, look at the back label and add the DHA and EPA amounts; the total will tell you how much beneficial fatty acid you're getting.

I've found the Nordic Natural and Eskimo Oil brands of fish oil are best. I recommend at least 1,000 milligrams a day, and possibly more based on your mood issues. Check with your doctor before you start taking fish oil supplements since they can interact with some medications.

7 TRUST YOUR GUT AND TAKE CARE OF IT

NO ONE ARGUES against eating a healthy diet, the benefits go beyond what we traditionally have believed.

THE STORY

Georgia was a 70 year-old-woman who I had been treating for years. She suffered from fibromyalgia, depression, and weight gain. Every time I would see her, we would discuss diet and exercise and their importance in her ability to feel better. She had a tough time adhering to either.

She moved out of town, and I did not see her for three years. Recently, she came to see me for a full exam. She had lost ten pounds, her depression was gone, and so was her fibromyalgia. What had she done?

When she moved, she finally followed my advice and adopted a Mediterranean-style diet and joined a gym. She was able to get her excess weight off and keep it off, and she started feeling happy and no longer suffered from pain.

Experts and Evidence

I knew the Mediterranean diet was a good one based on epidemiologic studies.[1] After Georgia came to see me, I started to wonder why the diet worked so well, and that led me to an interesting discovery. One of the main reasons the diet is successful is because it fosters healthy gut bacteria. These are bacteria that line your intestines and help in the process of digestion. The population of gut bacteria, also known as the microbiome, is now considered an organ unto itself. The microbiome influences behavior, the immune system, cancer and heart disease risk, brain development, metabolism, and obesity in addition to overall inflammation.[2] When Georgia started eating healthy, she improved her microbiome and reduced her inflammation thus eliminating her pain.

There are many studies showing those eating the traditional, high fat, low fiber, Western diet have disrupted gut flora. The bacteria in the gut are essential for normal metabolism. They digest food and help to produce energy, vitamins and essential nutrients. What happens if they are disrupted is the mucosa, the protective barrier of the intestine, can break down. This increases the permeability of the intestines and allows bacteria and toxins to leak out. One of these bacteria-derived toxins is a part of the cell wall known as lipopolysaccharide, or LPS. This can trigger an inflammatory response and can lead to depression. This effect has been illustrated in animal models where LPS has been given, and the animal then exhibits depression. The induced depression is reversed by antidepressants. Equally fascinating is in addition to the depressive response, there may be an autoimmune response to serotonin (our feel good hormone) that has been associated with fatigue.

It is the high fat diet that increases the likelihood of increased intestinal permeability, also known as "leaky gut." The strongest influence on microbial behavior is a long term, habitual diet. When people eat a plant-based diet rich in vegetables, fruits and fermented food, the intestinal wall heals and there is no more leakage of LPS, and their inflammation goes down.

The College of William and Mary conducted a psychological study of students. They studied those who scored high on the anxiety and neuroticism scale.[3] They found students who regularly ate fermented foods did not show any signs of anxious behavior. This demonstrates the gut microbiome is at least partially responsible as a cause of anxiety.[4]

Studies have found animals put in situations which peaked their anxiety were less likely to be anxious if they had healthy gut flora. Those with unhealthy flora suffered extreme anxiety. One study linked it to fat mice. Scientists painted skinny, anxious mouse poop on their front legs. The fat mice licked it off, essentially doing a fecal transplant on themselves. The result, the fat mice lost weight and became anxious.[5] There have also been many studies showing lean mice become obese when bacteria from obese human individuals are transplanted into their gut. An experiment was done on mice that were genetically predisposed to become fat. They were housed in the same cage with thin mice. Mice eat each other's poop (just a disgusting mouse fact). When the mice who were genetically programmed to be fat ate the poop of the thin mice, they did not get fat! They had done a successful stool transplant on themselves. Healthy bacteria were restored in their gut, keeping them from getting fat, and preventing them from following their genes.[6]

The gut-brain connection is now being widely studied, and we still have much to learn. It is entirely possible in the future we will be treating obesity, behavioral, and mood disorders with probiotics and even possibly fecal transplants. In the meantime, improve your mood and overall well-being by boosting your good bacteria and giving them an environment where they can thrive and survive.

You can do this by eating a healthy, clean diet rich in prebiotics that fertilize the flora. Foods that help include asparagus, beans, artichokes, garlic, root vegetables and other foods high in fiber. In addition, fermented foods are a natural source of probiotics. Probiotics are *organisms* or *bacteria*. These include yogurt, kefir, kimchi and sauerkraut. Avoiding antibiotics and food treated with antibiotics whenever possible is also important. Antibiotics kill and alter gut bacteria, upsetting the balance of the microbiome.

You can also take probiotics in a pill, liquid, powder—and even a vaginal suppository form. There are a huge number of brands and types to choose from.

Look for the type of bacteria they contain. The best probiotics contain multiple types and large numbers. The one I recommend most often is vsl#3 taken twice daily. This is a medical grade probiotic that contains eight strains in amounts that go from 112.5 billion to 900 billion. The strains are:

- Bifidobacterium longum
- Bifidobacterium infantis
- Lactobacillus acidophilus
- Lactobacillus plantarum
- Lactobacillus paracasei
- Lactobacillus bulgaricus
- Streptococcus thermophilus

It is key you know how to store the probiotics. Some, such as vsl#3, need to be refrigerated. If they are not stored properly they will die, and you will have an expensive bunch of dead organisms that won't do you any good.

Of course, if you do not change unhealthy eating habits, the probiotics won't help anyway. They need to enter an environment that will help them to live and multiply for your benefit.

EXERCISE WILL BOOST YOUR BACTERIA

Of the myriad benefits of exercise, one which is seldom noted, is that it is a natural and effective way to boost your good bacteria and keep them diversified.[7] It is something you can do every day . . . .

Exercise is an excellent way to keep the microbiome healthy. There are some promising results in athletes showing this phenomenon. Forty professional rugby players in Ireland were studied in comparison to normal weight and overweight non-athletes. The athletes had greater diversity of bacteria and healthier guts than the non-athletes.

Of course, the athletes ate a healthier, high protein diet, which may explain some of the results. The next logical question: what would be seen in non-athlete exercisers compared to those who do not exercise? Fortunately, a recent study arrived at an answer.

This study looked at 104 men and women between the ages of 18 and 45. Researchers compared those who were sedentary to those who exercised on average three to five hours a week. In those who exercised, there was a four-fold increase in good bacteria, which boosts the immune system. These findings were more pronounced in women.[8]

HOW DOES EXERCISE DO THIS?

Exercise increases the release of anti-inflammatory chemicals known as cytokines and myokines. It also increases the production of short chain fatty acids that enhance bacteria that produce butyrate. Butyrate reduces the risk of colon cancer, and reduces the release of the inflammatory LPS, which we mentioned earlier. It also boosts immunity by inducing the production of special regulatory T cells in the gut.[9]

CAN EXERCISE OVERRIDE UNHEALTHY EATING?

There is hope that it may be possible to override an occasional dietary splurge by maintaining a healthy exercise regimen. There was a study of mice that found when mice were exercised, they still had healthy guts despite a high fat diet.[10] Studies in humans are pending.

A REAL KILLER....

One food you think might be healthy can be deadly to your gut bacteria: artificial sweeteners. Discovered completely by accident in 1879, the original sweetener known as saccharin was found when a chemistry research assistant at Johns Hopkins Hospital was working on finding a food preservative. He accidentally spilled the new compound on his hands. When he went home that night, he picked up a dinner roll and noticed its incredible sweetness (I know it's gross, but he didn't wash his hands after the spill!). He realized he was onto something and named this new compound after the Latin word *saccharum*, which means sugar.[11]

Since that time, there have been many new sweeteners introduced to the market, often with much press and fanfare. Each of these chemicals has been heralded as nothing short of a miracle: your food and drinks sweet and tasty yet with no increase in calories! What an easy way to lose weight and keep blood sugars low! Some doctors and dietitians even recommend them. The catch? Yes, sadly, there is just a little catch: they do not have the desired effect. Ironically, they increase glucose intolerance by altering the bacteria and doing the opposite of what they were designed to do! They *actually cause weight gain* and increase blood sugar. It would be best to avoid them if you want to promote a healthy microbiome[11] and overall health, for that matter.

Sorry to be a buzz-kill for all you diet soda drinkers.

Coffee, Chocolate, Lemon Balm,
and Mushrooms

8 Fun Foods You Didn't Know Were Healthy

Coffee

THERE ARE CERTAIN foods and drinks that have gotten a bad rap over time. Coffee is one of them. I have to come clean and confess I am hooked on it. I started drinking coffee after school in junior high with my mom and her friends. I felt so grown up as I regaled them with my tales of woe, and explained how I was never going back to school.

Obviously, I did go back to school, and I kept drinking coffee. Over the years, I have kept up with studies about this tasty brew since I have a vested interest in making sure it is okay for me to drink. There was a bit of a scare in 1981 when an article in the *New England Journal of Medicine* described an increased risk of pancreatic cancer associated with coffee drinking. It turns out the study was biased. The researchers had matched the patients with cancer to control patients that were in the hospital for gastrointestinal problems. Those patients were told NOT to drink coffee even though many had been regular coffee drinkers, and that made it look like coffee was a factor in pancreatic cancer. Fortunately, it is not.[1]

Since that time, there have been many studies looking at coffee and health. The benefits are many. Let's start at the top and work our way down.

THE BRAIN

The most impressive effects of coffee are seen in the brain. Many of us find it is what we need to get going and prepare for the day. Of course there is the ritual of drinking that first cup, but most importantly, it snaps us into focus. It has many other benefits beyond the "alertness" factor particularly when it comes to neurologic disease. Coffee has been associated with a lower risk of Parkinson's disease. However, the protective effect was only with caffeinated coffee. Those who drink it are anywhere from 32 to 60 percent less likely to develop the disease. It has also been found to improve motor function in those who have Parkinson's.[2]

Coffee also has a protective effect against Alzheimer's disease. The results of a large, long-term study known as the Cardiovascular Risk Factors, Aging and Dementia (CAIDE) study found coffee drinkers had a 65 percent decreased risk of developing the disease.[3]

Coffee has been associated with a decreased risk of depression in women. For those who drank four or more cups a day, their risk of depression was reduced by 20 percent. A study done at Harvard found those who drink two to four cups a day decrease their risk of suicide by 50 percent.[4]

Coffee drinkers are also able to focus when tired. After drinking a cup, their reaction times, reasoning ability and attention improve.[5]

A combination of 11 studies found two-to-six cups a day was associated with a lower risk of stroke, about 20 percent, when compared to nondrinkers.[6]

Multiple sclerosis is a disease that affects 2.3 million people worldwide. An analysis of two case-control studies done at Johns Hopkins University found there was a link between coffee consumption and MS. The researchers found participants who did not drink coffee in the year prior to the onset of symptoms were 1.5 times more likely to develop MS when compared to those who drank four cups of coffee a day. In this case, it appears caffeine is neuroprotective.[7]

Finally, the very large Nurses Health Study found women who consumed about six cups of coffee a day had a 21 percent decreased risk of developing tinnitus or ringing in the ears.[8]

THE HEART OF THE MATTER

Although coffee can increase blood pressure when used sporadically and can cause the heart to race if one overindulges, researchers have found moderate, long-term coffee consumption of three to five cups a day lowers the risk of heart disease.[9] This is probably due to the phytochemicals in coffee that reduce inflammation, the process that contributes to heart disease.

THE PANCREAS AND LIVER

Drinking six to seven cups of either caffeinated or decaffeinated coffee a day was found to reduce the risk of developing type 2 diabetes by 23 to 50 percent. Controlled studies have found with the consumption of each cup, the risk decreases by seven percent up to five cups a day.[10]

Coffee decreases the risk of alcohol-related cirrhosis by up to 80 percent in those who drink four or more cups a day. It also reduces the risk in those with nonalcoholic fatty liver disease.[11]

CANCER

Drinking two cups of coffee a day reduces the risk for liver cancer by 40 percent.[12] Four to five cups a day reduces the risk for endometrial cancer by 20 percent.[13] It reduces the risk of lung cancer in those who smoke.[14] It may also reduce the risk for melanoma and basal cell cancers of the skin.[15]

A study of over 5000 people with colorectal cancer who were compared to 4000 people without cancer found those who drank two and a half cups of coffee a day had a 50 percent lower risk of colorectal cancer compared to those who did not drink coffee. Interestingly, it did not matter whether it was caffeinated or decaffeinated.[16]

DEATH(!)

Drinking coffee significantly reduces the risk of premature death by 20 percent in men and 26 percent in women.[17]

IN SUMMARY

Why is coffee so beneficial? It is probably due to the fact it is packed with antioxidants that keep us healthy. It also increases our sensitivity to insulin, which may account for its positive effect on the brain.

Aside from the potential cardiac issues mentioned above, the other downside to coffee is what it may do to your sleep if you drink it near bedtime. The other potential problem for regular drinkers is what happens if you stop. You will get a whopping headache. I make sure that never happens!

We would be remiss if we didn't remind you that, while coffee itself has no calories, the calories can certainly add up when you drink fancy coffee drinks. A 20-ounce Mocha Frappuccino at Starbucks is 500 calories and has an astounding 79 grams of sugar.

Finally, if you brew coffee at home, drip filtered coffee is fine. Coffee contains oils known as terpenes, which if left in the brew can raise LDL or "bad" cholesterol levels. The old-fashioned percolator coffee and the new-fashioned French press coffee both make unfiltered coffee that may increase cholesterol levels. [18] You might want to drink these types of coffee in moderation if cholesterol is an issue for you.

Chocolate

Next up is another one of my favorites. Chocolate has a deep and "rich" history. It goes back as far as 1900 BC, to Mesoamerica. The Aztecs thought the cacao seeds were a gift from the gods. They believed it was an aphrodisiac and gave strength when consumed.

For those of us in modern times, chocolate is revered for its taste, avoided due to its calories, and has been described as a guilty pleasure. However, for the last several years, chocolate has been touted as a health food. Chocolate contains the following:

- Tryptophan and serotonin—naturally occurring chemicals that give us a sense of well-being
- Caffeine—a stimulant
- Xanthines—increases wakefulness
- Theobromine—a stimulant that increases blood flow and acts as a cough suppressant
- Anadamide—activates pleasure receptors in the brain
- Pheynlthylamine—stimulates the release of dopamine, associated with feelings of pleasure
- Flavanols—plant or phytonutrients that act as powerful antioxidants that boost blood flow and act as a mild analgesic (i.e. pain reliever).

The question: Looking at the above ingredients, is chocolate really healthy?

The answer: If eaten in moderation and in its pure form, there are many benefits. Let's start at the top again.

THE BRAIN

Research at Harvard Medical School found seniors who drank two cups of hot cocoa a day for a month had improved blood flow of the brain and memory. It only worked with chocolate that contained high levels of antioxidants, otherwise known as dark chocolate.[19]

A Canadian study of over 44,000 people found people who ate chocolate were 22 percent less likely to suffer a stroke than those who did not. They were also 46 percent less likely to die as a result.[20] Chocolate also makes us feel good. It boosts endorphins and it can create a similar effect to cannabis, but in a small way, because to make a real psychotropic impact an average size person would have to eat 25 pounds. So, the reason it may perk us up and make us happy is probably due to the taste, texture and the overall experience.[21]

THE HEART

Chocolate lowers the risk of developing heart disease by a full one third in those who eat it regularly. In a study of 21,000 people from

Norfolk, England that took place over 11 years, of those who were in the top level of chocolate consumption, 12 percent developed cardiovascular disease compared to 17.4 percent who did not eat chocolate.[22]

A study of 470 elderly men found cocoa reduced the risk of cardiovascular death by 50 percent over a 15-year period.[23] Another study revealed eating chocolate five times a week lowered the risk of disease by 57 percent.[24] Yet another study found eating chocolate two or more times a week decreased the risk of calcified plaque in the arteries by 32 percent.[25]

Chocolate improves some of the risk factors for cardiovascular disease. The flavanols in dark chocolate stimulate the lining of blood vessels to relax, and in doing so reduces blood pressure. Cocoa powder decreases LDL cholesterol in men and increases their HDL, or "good" cholesterol.[26]

THE SKIN

The flavanols in chocolate can protect against sun damage of the skin. In a study of 30 people, the time required to develop redness doubled after eating one third of a two-ounce dark chocolate bar every day for 12 weeks.[27]

AS IF CHOCOLATE ISN'T WONDERFUL ENOUGH . . .

If you are in a movie, concert or play and feel like you have to cough, I have a tip for you. I mentioned earlier chocolate contains theobromine which acts as a cough suppressant. If you take a small square of dark chocolate and let it melt on your tongue, it will stop your cough for about an hour. Keep some in your purse or pocket and give it a try the next time you have to fight the urge.

IN SUMMARY

Chocolate in moderation is healthy. It is important to eat a small square (1.5 oz.) with 70 percent organic cocoa or higher. The healing power is in the cocoa content.

Lemon Balm: A Natural Treatment for Herpes

Ninety percent of Americans experience at least one cold sore in their lifetime. Forty percent have recurring infections. That is why a natural, inexpensive remedy would be a wonderful thing to have.[28] The herpes virus is responsible for causing cold sores *and* genital herpes. Generally, the herpes virus 1 (HSV 1) causes cold sores and herpes virus 2 (HSV 2) causes genital herpes.

Lemon balm, also known as *Melissa Officinalis,* is a great natural treatment for these viruses. The plant is easy to grow outside and can be grown inside as well. There are properties of the plant that explain its therapeutic effect. The leaves contain plant substances called tannins and terpenes that give the plant its antiviral effects. They also contain eugenol, which helps with pain and discomfort and kills bacteria.

Studies have shown topical lemon balm cream and ointments can heal cold sores. In one study of 66 people, lemon balm cream was applied and patients experienced significant decreased redness and swelling after two days. Unfortunately, the cream did not affect the scabbing and discomfort.[29]

A series of impressive studies were done in Germany. The results showed when lemon balm was used to treat a *first time* infection of HSV 1, not a single recurrence was found. In addition, it reduced healing time of both genital and oral herpes.[30]

HOW CAN LEMON BALM BE USED?

Lemon balm can be found in ointments and creams. Soaking a cotton ball in lemon balm extract and dabbing it on the cold sore can also be very effective. Lemon balm tea can be used as a facial or body wash or soak. Lemon balm soft gels can be taken orally. Preparations are relatively inexpensive, and if you want to be even more natural, you can grow the plant in your garden and make your own teas and extracts.

WHEN SHOULD LEMON BALM BE USED?

For those plagued with cold sores, we recommend patients apply lemon balm nightly to their lips to prevent them. It feels good, works well and keeps the lips from getting chapped. For outbreaks, we suggest applying the cream or ointment four to five times a day. For genital herpes, put the extract or tea in a bath and soak. It will be soothing at the very least, and many people find it helps with the intensity and duration of symptoms. It is worth a try, and fortunately there have been no reported side effects.

Magical Medicinal Mushrooms

Whenever I mention mushrooms to my patients, they start to giggle. They remember the psychedelic mushrooms of the '60s. The mushrooms I am talking about are medicinal. They are the same ones used in cooking, but for my purposes I recommend the concentrated form of capsules. Mushrooms are classified as vegetables, but they are not really plants. They are fungi. And they are amazing!

Many of them can be used to detoxify contaminated environments. They have enzymes that break down plant fiber. These enzymes also reduce hydrocarbons and other manufactured toxins. Once they have finished their job, the pollutants can be used as fertilizer. What mushrooms do for the environment, they also do for the body; they are great detoxifiers. They also feed the microbiome we talked about earlier, acting as prebiotics. As we explained, prebiotics are defined as a nondigestible food component that promotes the growth of beneficial microorganisms in the intestines. Asparagus, onions and leeks are good examples (not to be confused with probiotics, which are live microorganisms that, when administered in adequate amounts, confer a health benefit to the host).

Research has shown Reishi and Turkey Tail mushrooms boost the immune system, balance the microbiota, resulting in improved digestion, and also help with weight loss.[31]

Because mushrooms are such great detoxifiers, it is important that when you eat them or use them in a medicinal blend, they are organic and have been grown in a controlled environment. Otherwise, you may end up consuming them with all the toxins they are in the midst of breaking down.

For that reason, I recommend a particular brand of medicinal mushrooms. It is called Host Defense, by Paul Stamets, the "mushroom king." He has been studying mushrooms for decades and has perfected his blends. You can find out more about him and his mushrooms at fungi.com. His products are sold online and at Whole Foods.

I recommend mushrooms to my patients for a whole host of reasons. There are several varieties that include the aforementioned Turkey Tail, Reishi, Maitaki, Shitaki, Cordyceps, and Lion's Mane. I'll briefly describe the benefits of each. If you want them all and then some, there is a blend of 17 mushrooms called MyCommunity, available commercially.

REISHI

The use of this mushroom goes back centuries. It was called the "Mushroom of Immortality." It has many positive effects, including immune-enhancing properties. It is also helpful in cancer treatment, disrupts viral illness, inhibits bacteria and improves liver function. It has been found to lower blood pressure, improve allergies, act as an anti-inflammatory, and help to reduce stress and insomnia. This mushroom has the ability to calm tension, and is why some say it has the power to extend life.[32]

MAITAKE

This mushroom is often called "The Hen of the Woods" because that is what it looks like. Its beneficial effects are numerous. In Asia it is traditionally used to treat diabetes and high blood pressure. However, it may help with many other problems, one of which is improving fertility in those with polycystic ovarian syndrome. These women have difficulty getting pregnant due to hormonal issues.[33]

There are medications available to help; however, mushrooms are nutritious and without side-effects. They can be used alone or to augment medical treatment.

The maitake mushroom has an antitumor effect in bone marrow tumor colony formations and reduces toxicity of some chemo-therapeutic agents. It enhances immune activity against bladder cancer cells, and it reduces inflammation in inflammatory bowel disease. In a small group of cancer patients, the Maitaki mushroom was found to induce tumor regression, and it improved symptoms in half the patients.[34]

SHIITAKE

Shiitake mushrooms are commonly seen on restaurant menus because they are so tasty. But they also have tremendous healing properties. They are rich in B vitamins, selenium, copper, zinc, manganese and vitamin D. In addition, they are an excellent source of iron that is easy for the body to access.

As far as overall health effects, they reduce the risk of cardio-vascular disease by protecting blood vessels. These mushrooms block harmful molecules from binding to the vessels and causing them damage. This cellular injury is responsible for the process of atherosclerosis, otherwise known as hardening of the arteries, a condition which increases the risk for a heart attack. In addition, they also have antiviral and anticancer properties.[35]

CORDYCEPS

Cordyceps is a weird little fungus. It grows on caterpillars in the Himalayan Mountains. It has been used as a tonic in Chinese medicine to improve energy. It has been found to improve blood flow, and it helps breathing by opening airways. It prevents bacterial and viral infections, reduces cholesterol and increases sperm production both in quantity and quality.

I remember being introduced to this mushroom in capsule form when I was training with Dr. Andrew Weil. I was shocked at the energy-producing effect it had on me, and for that reason, I often recommend it to my patients. It is a great energy booster in the afternoon when people tend to get sleepy, and it does not interfere with sleep at night.

TURKEY TAIL

This mushroom is found all over the Pacific Coast here in the United States. It lives on fallen hardwood trees and branches. It's so named because it looks just like a turkey tail. This is a mushroom I recommend to all my patients with cancer or who have a family history of cancer. Studies done first in Japan and now in the United States have found when used in combination with chemotherapy, it enhances the therapeutic effect. It also reduces the side effects of treatment. It has been found to be beneficial in the treatment of breast, cervical, lung, esophageal, skin and stomach cancers.[36] Studies are ongoing by the National Institutes of Health.

In addition to the above, Turkey Tail mushrooms have strong antiviral properties against viruses known to cause cancer. The two it's known to fight are Human Papilloma Virus which causes cervical cancer and the Hepatitis C virus that causes liver cancer. The same study suggested it may inhibit HIV as well.[37]

THE STORY

Ten years ago, Helen, a 58-year-old woman, came to see me at my clinic. She had been diagnosed by biopsy with a rare skin cancer, Merkel cell carcinoma. It is a neuroendocrine tumor (stemming from the nerve and hormone system). Deviously, it appeared as a painless red bump on her left index finger that was growing quickly and deeply. As you can imagine, Helen was pretty upset ("freaked out" were her words) when she found out. Due to scheduling and insurance issues she and her doctor made a plan to have the whole tumor removed a month later at the University of Washington. I prescribed four capsules of the Host Defense Stamets 7 blend (containing Royal Sun Blaze, Cordyceps, Reishi, Maitake, Lion's Mane, Chaga and Mesima) in the morning, and four more Lion's

Mane capsules in the evening before meals. I chose the extra Lion's Mane because she also had back pain, and it is known to help with nerve problems. She took them faithfully for a month. Then, she had her tumor removed; all seemed to have gone well. Another month later, I received a call from her surgeon. He wanted to know what I had done for her prior to the surgery. I told him all I had done was start her on the mushrooms. He proceeded to tell me that between the time of the biopsy and the tumor removal, all the cancer cells had died. He believed the mushrooms had something to do with the tumor cell death. Helen has continued to take her mushroom capsules and has remained in remission for ten years!

Experts and Evidence

LION'S MANE

Lion's Mane looks just like its name and is delicious and nutritious. When sautéed, it tastes a lot like lobster and contains 20 percent protein.

The use of Lion's Mane mushrooms in the treatment of Merkel cell carcinoma is being explored. Merkel cell is a tumor that is difficult to treat, and one of the big challenges of this cancer is it has often spread by the time it is discovered. Medicinal mushrooms, in particular, Lion's mane, has proven to be an effective treatment for some patients [38]. It certainly has been for my patient. After remaining cancer free on the mushroom capsules for ten years, she is utterly convinced they've saved her life. For other patients with this kind of tumor, there is no harm in using it. There are no side effects, and it is considered a healthy food.

Lion's Mane mushrooms also protect the nervous system. There are studies in rats showing when a main nerve in the foot of the animal is crushed, it grows back when the rat is treated with the mushrooms. [39]

Lion's Mane has been found to help with mild cognitive impairment as well. In a study done in 2009, 30 subjects with Alzheimer's disease were given Lion's Mane capsules of 250 mgs three times a day for 16 weeks. Compared to the placebo, those given the mushrooms improved significantly. Four weeks after the study was stopped, they deteriorated. The mushrooms only worked to improve their memory while they were taking them.[40]

Finally, a study of 30 postmenopausal women found those who ate Lion's Mane cookies versus those who ate cookies without it showed less anxiety and depression, and they were able to concentrate better![41]

9 What Women Want When it Comes to Sex

IT'S NO SECRET sex makes most people happy. Studies verify it, proving having sex about once a week is optimal for happiness for most people. In addition, studies also show sexually active people not only are happier, but they live longer, too. We've put together some important information to help you have better sex, and thus enjoy a longer, better life. [1]

On television, we see Viagra commercials aimed at men on a daily basis. It is helpful to men, but is there such a thing as Viagra for women?

Experts and Evidence

In 1998 Viagra rose out onto the prescription drug scene as the answer for men with erectile dysfunction problems. It has revolutionized sex for older men. It has also been studied in women with mixed results. A study of over 200 women done by Dr. Laura Berman and her team found 69 percent of women with normal estrogen and testosterone levels experienced improved sensation after taking 50 to 100 mgs of Viagra.

Another study done on women taking antidepressants (which can dull the sexual response and libido) found Viagra improved women's experience by 72 percent versus. 27 percent by placebo.[2]

Unfortunately, women experience similar side effects to men that include headache, nasal congestion, flushing, nausea and visual symptoms.[3] While it is clear Viagra can help some women, the side effects may be enough to keep women from trying it. There is another option: "Scream Cream." It is a mix of Viagra, Aminophylline and L-Arginine. These are all compounds that dilate blood vessels. The cream is made by a compounding pharmacy. It is applied an hour before sexual activity to the clitoral area. It helps to improve sensitivity and sexual function. It works splendidly for most of my patients. There are no side effects, and we have noted no long-term adverse effects.

THE STORY

Sylvia is a 65-year-old woman who suffered a stroke 3 years ago. She was left with some weakness on her left side. Although she regained some of her strength, she developed a mild depression commonly seen in stroke survivors, which did improve with the antidepressant Celexa. She and her husband had always enjoyed a healthy sex life; however, the antidepressant dulled her sensation and it was hard for her to achieve orgasm. She also noted increasing vaginal dryness was causing her discomfort. To improve her sensation, I prescribed Viagra cream, which has been available as a prescription for the last few years at our compounding pharmacy. For the vaginal dryness I had her start using vaginal estriol mini-inserts, which she started using every other night. She applied the cream to her clitoral area about 45 minutes before engaging in intercourse. Her vaginal dryness improved and her sensation returned. In fact, things started going so well she and her husband had a "second honeymoon" in Hawaii.

They were having so much fun in bed one night that her screams of ecstasy were mistaken for someone being brutally attacked, and the next thing they knew, they had concerned hotel security banging on their door fearing she was being harmed. They both became quite embarrassed, but explained they were just having fun—and coined the term "Scream Cream" for *her* Viagra!

WE WANT TO MAKE SURE YOU ARE SCREAMING FOR THE RIGHT REASON . . . .

Scream cream can definitely spice up your sex life. However, if you suffer from vaginal dryness you may not find it much fun. Twenty to forty percent of women in midlife and beyond suffer from this condition (also known as "vaginal atrophy" in the medical world, but we prefer "dryness" to this rather unkindly medical designation). [4, 5] After menopause, due to lack of hormones, the tissues of the vagina become dry, and sex is often painful as a result. There are many treatments for this. I will share the ones I have found to be most successful for my patients.

If your doctor determines it is safe for you to use hormones, vaginal estriol is an effective treatment. It is a very weak form of estrogen and is relatively safe.[6] It is often used in women who have been treated for breast cancer. I prescribe it as a mini vaginal insert in a low dose (0.5 mgs) that women use every other night. They are made by the compounding pharmacy. If your testosterone level is low, it can be added as well. This can improve your libido and you will find yourself having more fun than you have had in ages!

For a non-hormone solution, I recommend vitamin E vaginal suppositories made by Carlson. There are many studies showing they work and have no side effects. Carlson also makes fish oil capsules. Don't get them mixed up like one of my friends did! She inserted the fish oil by mistake. She was in horror at the time but, needless to say, later, we got a good laugh out of that one!

Finally, there is something else I recommend for dryness. It is called V-Magic. It is used on the vulvar area, which we know can become dry as we age. It consists of olive oil, avocado oil, beeswax, sea buckthorn and organic honey.[7] The combination is healing and soothing. Although it is designed for the vulvar area, many of my patients have actually used it for cuts, chapped lips and an abundance of irritated areas with great success.

AND FOR WOMEN WHO HAVE DISCOMFORT FOR ANOTHER REASON . . . .

Since Viagra is a powerful vasodilator, it has been explored for use in menstrual cramps, and it seems to work. A study conducted by Penn State College recruited 25 women to administer 100 mgs of Viagra vaginally. They rated their pain over a four-hour period. Those given Viagra were twice as likely to note relief as compared to those who were given a placebo. There were no side effects noted in either group.[8] Since the Viagra vaginal suppositories are not available commercially, I have been prescribing the compounded version. It has worked extremely well and has not caused any adverse effects. If you are one of those women who has been incapacitated by your periods due to pain, there is no longer a need to suffer.

As I stated earlier, a compounding pharmacy is needed for the above prescriptions. You need to discuss the possibility of using these with your doctor. The local pharmacy I use is Wellness Compounding Pharmacy www.wellnessformyhealth.com/. You may find your own local favorite by going to www.findacompounder.com.

THE IMPACT OF HOW WE FEEL ON THE ENJOYMENT FACTOR

So far, we have spoken about the physicality of how to enjoy sex. One of the things we as women know is much of our enjoyment has to do with how we feel about our partner; we need to feel comfortable and cared for. In other words, our most powerful sex organ is our brain.

But what's going on inside *men*? How do men view us, and what would be the best approach for us to start and/or maintain a healthy relationship, sexually and otherwise?

THE STORY

Fay is a 40-year-old woman who grew up in a family of all women, the eldest of four sisters. Her father left when she was a baby, and as she grew up, she was often left to care for her siblings when her mother was working. As a teenager and young adult, she had a very limited social life. She went to an all-girls high school. She attended a local college to be close to home. That is where she met and married her first boyfriend. She was head-over-heels for him. They married within six months of meeting, and she moved from her mother's house to his house.

Initially, things went great. The newlyweds were having fun getting to know each other. Sex was new and she was enjoying herself. Over time, they settled into a routine. They both worked full time. She did what she was used to doing growing up; she took responsibility for the lion's share of the family chores. She became overwhelmed. She started to resent her husband and became withdrawn from him. She was exhausted at night and sex, which had been fun and exciting, no longer appealed to her.

She came to see me as a patient. After some frank questioning, it turned out she had not discussed anything about her feelings with her husband. He was a very caring man who loved her and was totally unaware of how burdened she felt. Growing up with women, she had little experience speaking to men. I suggested she give it a try, and little by little, she opened up to him and started asking for help around the house and for time away together. He happily complied, and within about six months her life had improved, and they were enjoying each other both in and out of the bedroom.

Experts and Evidence

Fay's experience is not unique. I don't need to state the obvious, but I will. Men and women are very different. Sometimes (okay, a lot of the time) men baffle us. We are often afraid to approach them about what is bothering us. It would be nice to know what is going on in their heads when it comes to relationships. If we all had a big brother or good male friend to ask, life might be easier. How nice that we have one for you. Dave will give you a better understanding of the male perspective. It will help empower you to ask for what you want. By asking, you will not only improve your sex life, but your life in general.

A MAN'S LAST WORD ON RELATIONSHIPS

It's often said that first love is the sweetest and deepest. There's some truth to that—because we've never been hurt before. We give ourselves over innocently and completely, immerse ourselves in the intensely-wonderful, all-consuming flame. And it's perfect. Like a perfect flower. And it lasts! Until it withers and dies. It often takes years to get over our first love, and sometimes we never do. The next time we find love, we are less likely to fall with the same intensity. Pain is an excellent teacher.

You are probably like I am, no longer with your first love, yet you still remember that first love with some fondness and bitter-sweetness. Well, I just lied. Even all these years later, I'm still mostly just bitter. But not with her: with myself.

I was completely head-over-heels in love. Yet she wasn't particularly sweet; in fact, she was pretty demanding and selfish. She was often totally unreasonable and downright unkind. A classic example: She lived in the next town over, and sometimes we couldn't see each other for a couple of days. With my heart overflowing, I'd practically run toward her for our embrace.

"Oh no. Don't come over here and expect me to be all *overjoyed* to see you," she'd warn, eyes flashing, jaw clenched.

Shocked and hurt, I'd stop and plead, "Honey, what's wrong? What did I do?"

"*'What's wrong?' 'What did I do?'*" she'd mockingly retort. "Dave, if you don't even know, *I'm* not going to tell you."

But as I said, I'm not bitter towards her. That's who she was, and she was doing the best she could. I was with the wrong person, and—here's the kicker—even then I knew it, and I stayed. Far too long. That's why I look back on that relationship, more accurately on that younger iteration of myself, with bitterness.

Let my pain be your excellent teacher. If your person is treating you in a way that doesn't work for you, make some serious changes or get the hell out.

This brings me to my man's word on relationships: *ask.* That's right; I've boiled it down to a single word. This simple, one-syllable word applies to all romantic relationships, long-term or not, even to single people not yet in a relationship.

TAKE A CHANCE

Single people first. When you become interested in someone, take the scary chance and *ask.* Do it honestly and respectfully. You won't regret it; even if it ends up being a no-thanks, you'll still feel good about yourself for having been brave enough to go for it. And for every single time I've summoned up my courage and taken the chance and asked, no one has ever been mean to me.

Think about it from your own point of view for a moment. Someone approaches you respectfully and tells you they are interested in you. Would you not find that flattering? Even if for whatever reason you are unavailable or just not feeling that same type of attraction, it's still a great compliment to receive.

I'm going to give you something specific to say for your first time, because you're going to be petrified. This one is for someone you're only just seeing, that classic girl (or guy) on the train moment.

"Hi, I'm_____. I've been noticing you, and I've just got this strong feeling that I have to come over here and take a chance and introduce myself." At that point, the two of you will hopefully be able to strike up a conversation. Be sure to get a number.

If my "line" sounds stagey or contrived to you or doesn't quite fit your situation, then modify it, or dump it all together and come up with something that feels better. Honestly, it doesn't matter *what* you say; you've just got to say *something*. You may stammer a bit, and you may literally be shaking. That's okay. Stay strong and get through it. Remember, if you *don't* ask, it's a guaranteed no.

BE BRAVE

Women, you almost never have the courage to ask. We Americans tend to think of ourselves as so modern and liberated, and in many ways we are, but not when it comes to women asking men out. Some women will be interested in a man for weeks, months or even *years* and never let on, let alone approach him to let him know. The strategy many employ is to be nice and hope the guy makes his move.

Speaking from the male perspective, we are often too dense to decipher your subtle methods. We might like you independently, and we may eventually muster our courage to ask you out, but often we don't. So there you are waiting, hoping . . . and alone.

Honestly, most of us guys are easy. In other words, if you actually did let us know that you were interested, you'd suddenly become ten times more attractive to us. Not only because you would then become a real possibility, but also because to most, confidence is an attractant. (Men, note this last sentence also definitely applies to you.) *Ask.*

Okay. So now you've found your person, and you're in a relationship. You're off the market and the pressure's off. Is it perfect? No, of course not. You are both human, and you are flawed, so it can't be perfect. But it's probably going okay. Mostly. Ish.

But it's likely there are things you wish your person would do, or not do more of, or even do less of. And do you tell your person? No, you usually don't. You care about your person, and after all, it is going okay, and you certainly don't want to cause more friction or stress or, heaven forbid, a fight. And besides, you tell yourself, the timing isn't right just now. So, just like when you were single and had such a hard time asking, you say nothing and hope things get better on their own.

MEN ARE NOT MIND READERS

In this way, you're being like my first girlfriend: "Guess what I'm thinking, and then do what I want you to do." Your person likes you—your person wants you to like them back and wants to make you happy, but your person can't read your mind! Don't play that game. Instead, muster your courage and ask for what you want. This could easily be about sex. You may want more of *this,* and less of *that.* But it could really be about anything from laundry to disciplining the dog. Once again, you not asking gets you a guaranteed no. Not ever asking will get you a whole lot of no's, and will likely leave you unfulfilled, frustrated and even resentful.

Yes, asking for what you want makes you vulnerable and does risk confrontation. But this is *your* life with *your* special person! You deserve to be as happy together as you can possibly be, and that's not possible if you hold back and don't ask. If you do summon up the courage and ask, you have a real chance of making things better.

[Spoiler alert!] Romeo and Juliet literally died because of a lack of communication. You probably won't die if you don't ask for what you want, but you already know relationships are hard, and your not asking could snuff a good thing.

My last word on relationships? By now you already know it well, and I give you my word that it works: *ask.*

*The only way you get that fat off is to eat less
and exercise more.*

—JACK LALANNE

PART III
The Undiet (AKA the TEID DIET)

INTRODUCTION

For most of us, fitness is a struggle to attain. We are busy with work and family, and unfortunately workouts and healthy meal planning fall to the bottom of many of our to-do lists. That is why we felt it was important to devote this whole section to giving you tools that are easy to use and tips that are easy to follow to help you get in shape and stay there.

In Part III, you are being given your own personal trainer. I present to you my good friend and co-author, Dave Kahn. He is a certified personal trainer, competitive power lifter who holds a state record for lifting and is a nationally competitive West Coast Swing dancer.

You may not love what he has to say all the time, but the information is good; if you listen, you can learn great ways to attain fitness. Consider him your trainer in a book. Enjoy!

10 I WAS TOO FAT . . .

I WAS NOT fat. I was merely a "husky" kid. At least, that's what my mom insisted. To this day she sticks with that story. In truth, overweight, or fat, is exactly what I was. To give my mom some credit, I wasn't *obese*, but I was big enough to be self-conscious and unhappy about the way I looked, big enough to be teased occasionally by peers and family. In short, I was too fat.

I remember an older cousin, seeing that I had forgotten to zip up after the bathroom, asking, "Popped your pants, huh fatty?"

I was heaviest during my 12th and 13th years, about the worst possible time to be overweight for a kid. I was just starting to notice bodies—girls' especially, and here I was feeling ashamed of my own. Not that I was particularly conscious of this at first. Instead of facing the problem head on and taking steps to change, I just avoided it.

If you've never been heavy yourself, then perhaps this seems odd to you. How does one avoid the problem of being overweight when one is literally surrounded by it constantly? It's counter-intuitive that

I could have had any degree of success if avoiding my own physical truth was Plan A. But like I said, it wasn't a planned plan; it just kind of evolved into a de facto strategy.

It turned out I was pretty successful. I did three main things to keep myself (and others) away from my weight problem.

- I wore extra clothes. Lots of baggy sweaters, etc.
- I avoided the beach and pools (kids, even friends— or especially friends—can be exceptionally cruel).
- I avoided looking in the mirror.

Why share these embarrassing details? I've been there. I've been there, and I really didn't like it—or myself. The struggles I had are typical of anyone who is overweight or out of shape; I feel your pain, and I'm here to help.

A WAKEUP CALL

Even though extra weight often causes suffering and unhappiness, and of course eventually serious health issues, often it takes a specific incident to motivate actual change. We call this a threshold, or liminal, moment.

Robin had a patient named Freda whose story she shared with me. Freda is a woman who is in her 80s. Despite her good doctor's best effort urging her to eat healthier and start to slim down a bit (she was not morbidly obese), she resisted. Then one day, a friend sent her a picture she had taken of Freda while she had been visiting her. Freda was appalled at how heavy she looked. That was enough to do it. It took her some time and serious effort, but she has managed to shed, the extra pounds and she was feeling great.

TO START, WE HAVE TO TALK TECHNOLOGY

What's the coolest, most technologically advanced machine you know?

Think about this for a moment. Is it an AI robot, a fighter jet, the self-driving Google car? I'm still not over my amazing iPhone 5, which I hope to have forever and probably will, as long as I never make the mistake of updating.

Regardless of whatever machine you have in mind, I guarantee it has at least two major limitations.

1. Its parts wear out after a few years (or less) of continued use (especially if you accidentally drop it in the toilet).

2. Its application is limited because of its lack of adaptability. For example, you got rid of your flip phone because it no longer was able to do all that you expected it to do. No matter how much you love your GPS, it can't make you pancakes.

Wouldn't it be great to finally own a piece of equipment that . . .

* would fix *itself* if it got damaged?
* had an operating system (OS) that never needed updating, that always seamlessly dealt with new information without glitching or crashing?
* would actually be adaptive, so the more you used certain features, the more efficient and better those features would get?
* could accomplish many varied, complex and difficult tasks without major reprogramming?

Would you want that machine? Of course you would. Anyone and everyone would want it.

Well, you're in luck—if you order now, we can offer you such a machine at the low-low price of FREE! We call it:

Your amazing body. Even better, you already own it! Yes, we are all owners of the most durable, highly complex, highly adaptable machines in existence, bar none. (Note: unfortunately, no manual is included, but this book is a darn good start.)

The human body is a machine. It is an incredible, amazingly complex machine, but it is ultimately a machine.

It runs on fuel: food, which really means *calories.*

As we evolved as hunter-gatherers over millions of years, our bodies developed an amazing capacity to adapt to their environment.

- In situations where a lot of running was required, bodies got better at running, either at sprinting or distance running—or both.
- In situations where a lot of strength was required, bodies got stronger, either at repetitive motions or at huge bursts of strength—or both.
- In lean times, bodies adapted to survive on less, and in times of plenty, bodies adapted by storing excess food for later, for the lean times which were sure to return.

Of course, these amazing adaptations which supported our survival for millennia still work for us today. When people talk about *training*, either running, weight training or training for a sport, that's exactly what they're doing; they're training their bodies to adapt to specific stresses, and they get literally better, stronger, faster.

When I'm giving this information in the form of a talk in front of an audience, I actually play a bit of the old Six Million Dollar Man intro at this point. These days you can't even build a stretch of road for $6 million. The good news is these days, we actually do have the technology, and the vast majority of us can get in hugely better shape just by applying ourselves. (And for way less than the $6 million.)

So again, our bodies, being the super-amazing machines they are, adapt to how we train them. Our muscles literally get bigger and stronger from strength training. That's called *muscular hypertrophy.* (To pronounce this word correctly, place the stress on the "per.")

Muscular hypertrophy is one successful adaptation; storage of adipose tissue is another. When we put too much fuel into our machine, it doesn't waste it. Instead it converts into energy to be used for later (in times of famine, for example) in the form of adipose tissue, i.e.: fat. Fortunately, or perhaps unfortunately for many who could do with a curtailment of calorie intake, it's highly unlikely that America will ever see famine. As a society, we're stuck with feasting, and fattening ourselves continually.

BUT WAIT—BEFORE WE GET ANY FATTER, WHAT EXACTLY IS "FAT"?

Calling yourself or someone else "fat" is based on appearance; it's subjective. "Fat" to one may not be fat to another, or vice-versa.

"Overweight" and "obese" can be subjective terms, but they're also medical terms based specifically on one's Body Mass Index (BMI). BMI is the ratio of one's height to one's weight, and it's the most commonly used measure to evaluate someone's body shape.

BMI is a helpful measurement to give you a general idea of how you're doing, but don't take it too seriously if you're athletically built. At the peak of his bodybuilding career, Arnold Schwarzenegger, at 6 feet, 2 inches and ripped at 240 pounds, was *obese* according to the BMI scale. I'm in pretty decent shape, but I'm no Arnold; my BMI says that I'm only *overweight*.

There's a number of other options to measure how much fat you're carrying. Some are super-inconvenient and expensive, like hydrostatic weighing. That's the one where you get submerged in water. It is very accurate, but totally unrealistic for most people to do with any kind of ease or regularity. You can also have a bodyfat analysis on a dual-energy x-ray absorptiometry or DEXA scan. This is the same machine that's used to evaluate bone density. It takes about 20 minutes, is painless—but the price: $59 to $399![1] I'd recommend a standard bathroom scale. It's easy, simple and cheap. I'll talk more about how to use this common, time-tested tool in a bit.

If you want to get a little fancier, you can go with a scale that has a bioelectrical impedance option. These send a very low level of electric current through your body (we're talking AAA or even button batteries), and it has a little computer that measures the resistance in the current. Fat has a lower water content than muscle, so the current encounters more resistance if there's more muscle and gives the corresponding measurement. You also enter your height, and so you can get a more accurate assessment of your body composition. Recently these specialized scales have become much more common and inexpensive, and some are only around twenty dollars

AMERICA, YOU ARE FATTER THAN EVER, AND YOUR DIETING'S *NOT* HELPING!

We know we have a problem. We have the tools to fix it. We have the technology. We have tons of information and resources—this is America, dammit. Yet, the obesity epidemic in this country rages on.

The CDC (Centers for Disease Control and Prevention) and FRAC (Food Action Research Center) report that more than two-thirds— a full 68 percent—of Americans are either overweight or obese, with 32 percent registering in the obese category. This is more than ever before. These are crazy-high numbers! Just to give you some perspective, according to the World Health Organization's estimates, in the rest of the world, only about 13 percent are obese.[2]

Still, in America, we love to diet. The website bembu.com lists over 150 diet options. We spend about twenty billion dollar a year on them. All the choices and all the money doesn't change the fact that fighting fat through dieting simply does not help; the reality is most dieters fail miserably.

SOME HARD EVIDENCE OF THE FAILING FAT FIGHT

A comprehensive and rigorous study of 31 different diet programs was performed at the University of California, Los Angeles, to scientifically investigate the effectiveness of dieting. Their findings were consistent.

They found most diets will get you an initial five to ten percent weight loss, but it comes back. The majority of the dieters gained their weight back and then some. Only a very small number were able to keep their weight off. Their conclusion was that diets don't work. In fact, several studies indicate dieting is actually a consistent predictor of future weight gain![3]

A study published in the *American Journal of Public Health* reported more bad news for those struggling with their weight. This massive, long-term study encompassed eight years and had over 150,000 participants; it looked at the probability of an obese person attaining a normal body weight. Just 1 in 124 obese women was able to achieve normal weight. Just 1 in 210 men was able to achieve normal weight. In other words, a woman has a less than one percent chance of weight loss success, and a man has less than 0.5 percent chance. Clearly, we need to be doing something differently.[4]

Exercise, perhaps? We are not doing too well on that front either. The American Council on Exercise (ACE) reports that more than 50 percent of people who begin an exercise program discontinue within six months or less. A parallel statistic comes from a recent study from the IHRSA (International Health, Racquet & Sportsclub Association), the trade association that collects and analyzes data on the health and fitness industry: an amazing 67 percent of the people who have gym memberships *never* use them.

The good news? All these studies and statistics consistently verify one thing. *It is possible*—although it is no doubt challenging—*to get fit and stay fit.* The UnDiet (also known as the TEID DIET) may be that new approach that works for you.

WHAT IS THE TEID DIET?

"TEID" is diet spelled backwards; it is the UnDiet, which is simply smart eating and moving more, in that order. It's really that simple. There's no special club to join, no web site to subscribe to, no more books to buy, no meals, shakes or powders or pills to consume. Sure, there's a ton of plausible reasons you've been taught (and sold) so you'll take other approaches. What you need to do is *go back to basics.* How To?

HERE'S 12 QUICK, ECONOMICAL AND DOABLE THINGS. (THE *QEDS*)

1. NO MORE DIETING.

You need a different way.

2. GET NAKED AND GET ON THE SCALE.

Not only can it motivate you to change, it can empower you. Watching your numbers slowly (keyword: *slowly*) diminish and your body fat slowly subside feels good. The information and lack of avoidance helps you stay on track. I weigh myself on a digital scale every morning at the same time, before breakfast. It gives me a realistic picture of what I'm doing. If I'm a little over my goal weight then I'll cut back a bit. If I'm a little under, then I'll indulge a bit more that day. Depending on your preference, you may want to weigh yourself only once a week.

3. MOVE YOUR BODY MORE.

At least once a day for 30 minutes minimum, DO something. Our modern, much more sedentary lifestyle is a relatively new thing, and we're moving less than ever before. This is a big part of why, despite a lot of noise and billions of dollars spent, the obesity epidemic is drastically worsening. Today, many of us both work and play sitting down.

Start by taking walks, riding a bike for your errands, dancing, swimming, etc. Start taking the stairs, and park a little further away from the entrance.

4. STOP DRINKING YOUR CALORIES—DRINK WATER!

This one seems obvious, but most of us have trouble here.

It's hard to feel full after a can of soda, a glass of juice, a mug of beer or a caramel Frappuccino blended coffee. (Many of those coffee drinks are over 600 calories, and some are over 1,000!)

Let's do a little math here. You stop at the drive-by coffee hut each day on the way to work. It's easy to drop five dollars on a coffee drink and muffin/quick bite, and let's average the calories at a conservative 1,000 for the pair. Pencil it out at 50 weeks a year, times five days a week.

You've spent an unnecessary $1,250 consuming an unnecessary whopping 250,000 calories. Ending this one habit alone can be a huge game-changer in terms of your fitness.

Soda is a similar story. Public health researchers attribute over 184,000 global deaths each year to sugary drinks. In our country, consumption has increased significantly over the past 30 years. An astounding 50 percent of our population drinks them daily.

How do they kill so many people, though? Don't worry; it's only an *estimate*. Scientists looked at a huge amount of data, from 1980–2010, involving 611,971 people over 51 countries. They tracked 30 years of sugary drink consumption, and found sugary drinks caused 133,000 deaths from diabetes, 45,000 deaths due to cardiovascular disease and 6,450 deaths due to cancer.[5] Many experts consider sugary drinks to be the most fattening aspect of the modern diet.[6]

You might think you are being "good" by using a sugar substitute or drinking diet soda. However, as the *Yale Journal of Biology and Medicine* notes, "Several large scale prospective cohort studies found a positive correlation between artificial sweetener use and weight gain."[7] Diet soda has also been linked to an increased risk of stroke and heart attack![8]

Once again, keep it simple and be smart. Stick with water.

5. EAT CONSCIOUSLY. DISTRACTED EATING CAN BE A KILLER.

Stay away especially from "screen eating" —eating in front of a screen. A study published in the journal *Pediatrics* found watching TV is a major risk for obesity in children. It is not just the sedentary nature of watching that is the culprit.[9] It is the commercials that advertise sugary foods and drinks making them an object of desire that are a problem.

Distracted eating while watching also increases the amount of food eaten while in front of a screen. But matters are even worse; another study found TV watching in adults and children frees up the hands, making it easier to feed one's face.[10]

Researchers have also made a positive link between hours of TV watched and a reduced life expectancy due to sedentary behavior and overeating. They analyzed thousands of statistics and arrived at the conclusion that on average every single hour of TV viewed after the age of 25 reduces the viewer's life expectancy by 21.8 minutes.[11]

A screen is a screen. Eating in front of your laptop when you have Netflix, YouTube, or Facebook going (possibly simultaneously!) you are engaging in the behavior of distracted, unconscious eating, and this is not good for you.

Another place where it's common for people to eat unconsciously is the car. A recent study sponsored by Lytx, a global leader in video-based driver safety technology, found eating while driving was a close second to texting while driving in terms of danger. If you're eating or drinking while driving, you are 3.6 times more likely to be involved in a car crash than if you're not.[12] (Texting puts you at 4.6 times as likely.) Since it is not illegal to eat and drive, many people do not realize how risky it is. In addition to being downright dangerous, it is fattening. Somehow there is a mindset that calories consumed while eating in the car really don't count. Of course they do!

6. DON'T EAT LATE.

Breakfast, and eating early in general, can be a surprisingly important and effective tool in weight management. It's called calorie timing. Few people are aware of this amazing phenomenon; it feels like a trick or a gimmick, but it's real. It has to do with the body's natural circadian rhythms; our bodies actually want more fuel early and less fuel late. The old Chinese proverb recognized this years ago: "Eat breakfast like a king, lunch like prince and dinner like a pauper."

Modern scientists have proven this wisdom. A fascinating study was done to better understand how the human body uses calories over the course of a day. Ninety-three obese women were separated into two groups, the eat-early group and the eat-late group. Both groups were given a reduced calorie diet of the exact same foods and carefully monitored for cheating. The eat-early group ate a 700–calorie breakfast, a 500–calorie lunch, and just a 200–calorie dinner. The eat-late group's calorie intake was inverted. That is, they ate a 200–calorie breakfast, a 500–calorie lunch, and a 700–calorie dinner.

Members of both groups lost weight as expected, since all participants had significantly reduced their calorie consumption. However, the 12–week study showed that *when* they ate those calories had a big impact on weight loss. Those who ate the big breakfast lost an average of 17.8 pounds each and three inches off their waistline, while those in the big dinner group lost only 7.3 pounds and 1.4 inches off their waistline.[13]

The eat-early group lost more than *twice* as much weight!

7. DON'T EAT OUT AND STAY AWAY FROM EATING IN GROUP SITUATIONS.

Researchers at the Cornell University Food and Brand lab did a study on the getting-your-money's-worth hypothesis at meal time. They gave a discount to a group of diners at an all-you-can-eat pizza lunch buffet, and compared how much they ate to diners who paid full price. The full-price group ate 31 percent more pizza! The awareness of the additional cost significantly increased their food consumption.

Social eating is natural, and finishing the food on your plate is part of our national consciousness; it's what we've been trained to do as a culture. These values have been passed down for generations. Depending how old you are, you or members of your family were deeply affected by two major social-historical events that had a drastic impact on our country: the Great Depression and World War II. During the Depression, many families literally didn't have enough food to eat. To not finish your food was not only wasteful, it was also disrespectful and potentially harmful to your family. How dare you throw that food away?

Shortages on the Home Front during World War II were a real concern. America was sending not only her boys but also many of her resources and food overseas. There was a major wartime campaign to get people to support the war effort by not wasting our country's precious reserves. Posters reminded people to conserve, encouraging people to do their part by growing vegetables in a "Victory Garden." Another campaign exhorted citizens to clean their plates.[14] My parents were told to do their part and make a "Victory Plate," which meant eating every last scrap of the food in front of them. To not do so was unpatriotic. You love America, don't you? Eat!

How much we eat not only depends on our history and culture, but it also depends on with whom we're eating. Since we are social beings, we tend to eat more in group situations. And, we also eat more depending on how our dining partners look and how they eat. This has been proven.

The aforementioned researchers at the Cornell Food and Brand Lab monitored people's social eating in the same situation with the same foods, but with different eating companions. In one case, people sat down to a spaghetti dinner with a professional actress who wore a realistic disguise of an overweight prosthesis (i.e., "fat-suit"), and then served herself lunch. After observing her, male and female participants were asked to serve themselves pasta and salad to eat. In controlled variations of the study, the actress did not wear the fat-suit. The results demonstrated unequivocally that regardless of how the food was presented, participants served themselves and ate a larger amount of pasta—almost 32 percent more—when the actress was wearing the fat-suit than when she was not.[15]

These findings support a theory that when eating with or near an overweight person, you may be less likely to adhere to your own health goals. That is why it is important to think about how much you are going to eat *prior* to going to a restaurant.

Social eating can also challenge you in other ways. Many studies have shown the amount of food people eat is directly related to what others around them are eating. If your buddies are watching their intake, you will too. If others are splurging, odds are you will as well. It is something we humans are naturally programmed to do.[16]

That is why it is so important to stay aware and conscious of your food intake in these social situations; don't go to autopilot eating.

WHAT TO DO?

➡ Go in with a plan. One way to handle it is to eat a healthy meal just before you head out, and then explain you just ate and get a light salad. You'll still participate in the social eating, but not in the extra calories. (And you'll save some money, too!)

➡ Brush your teeth before you go out and plan to not eat. Sometimes just wanting to avoid having to do another cleaning can help you say no to food.

➡ Be aware that usually, no one truly cares if you eat or don't, or how much or how little you eat in these social situations.

8. PHONE A FRIEND (BUT BE CAREFUL ABOUT WHOM YOU CALL).

I'm going to tell you about my best buddy, Matt Murphy, who was my partner in overweight adolescence. One summer during junior high school, we decided to get serious and cut weight. Even then, the concept of the UnDiet was with us. We didn't sign up for a plan, even though there was a Jenny Craig center within walking distance and our folks would have paid. We didn't even buy a book. We went about it as simply as possible: We focused on eating less. We felt hungry, we wanted to eat more than we did, but we stuck together and supported each other, and it worked. We got thin together, and we have both been able to stay thin and fit ever since.

A scientific study backs up Matt's and my experience. It verifies working together with a friend to get fit makes for better success than going it alone. During the study, those who dieted with supportive friends did much better than those who dieted alone. Ninety-five percent of those with friends completed the initial dieting program compared to 76 percent who were solo, and at the time of the 10–month check-in, 66 percent with friends had kept the weight off, compared to just 24 percent who were solo—more than twice as much success with friends.[17]

Another massive, long-term study further verifies this. Researchers looked at data collected on obesity from more than 12,000 people over the last 30 years to try and figure out some of the mechanisms causing the obesity trend. Specifically, they looked at how obesity spreads and if it could be socially contagious. Are you more likely to gain weight if your friends, siblings, spouse and/or neighbors are gaining weight? In brief, the answer is *yes*.[18]

The link is strong. A person's chances of becoming obese increased by 57 percent if he or she had a friend who became obese. Among pairs of adult siblings, if one sibling became obese, the chance the other would become obese increased by 40 percent. If one spouse became obese, the likelihood that the other spouse would become obese increased by 37 percent.

An ally is a very good thing on this journey; by the same token, keep those who work against you at a distance when it comes to this part of your life.

9. THINK LONG-TERM.

Let's talk about holiday weight. Almost all of us put on a couple or few pounds during the winter holidays. We're surrounded by lots of goodies and parties with food. There is usually social pressure to eat pretty much everywhere, and many of us also reduce our physical activity in the winter. The weight gain is a very common occurrence. Let's assume we gain just two pounds.

Let's also assume come January, we (once again) fail to keep our New Year's resolution, and we don't go to the gym or start that step-aerobics class, and the weight stays on. Just two measly, little pounds—not much of a weight gain for the course of a whole year. Next year, the cycle repeats itself, and again you put on just two more pounds, and then again, just two pounds each following year. Multiply that by 20 years, and you've loaded up 40 extra pounds of fat. Thirty years, and you're up to 60 extra pounds.

10. SET A REASONABLE GOAL.

One pound a week is a reasonable goal.

To lose one pound in an entire week isn't much of a goal, but it is realistic and very doable.

Specifically, pick a day and time each week to weigh yourself for your weekly check-in.

Some weeks you're not going to make it. That's just the way it's going to be. That is not acceptable, so don't be complacent when that happens; get mad, stay committed and keep on. But *don't* beat yourself up and don't start playing catch-up. If you don't make the one pound weight loss that week, you don't "owe" two pounds the following week. Here's why: that's a quick road to feeling overwhelmed and to failure. Forgive yourself and move on. If on occasion you drop more than one pound in a week, that's not ideal, but at least it's in the right direction. The following week, dial it back just a tad and shoot for one pound again. Slow. Slow and steady.

Now consider this. You make your weekly goal of just one pound a week. In six months, you're down over 25 pounds, and that's real, controlled weight loss. In a year, you are down over 50 pounds. In just two years, you're down over 100.

Robin told me a good story that is a great example of this. She had a patient who was 225 pounds. She had gained the weight gradually over time. Her husband left her for another woman who was younger and thinner, and she was beside herself.

To deal with her angst, she started walking. She did a little to begin with, just a block. Then every day she increased it another block until eventually she was walking four miles a day.

She noticed she was losing weight and liked the way she felt. So, she started eating a healthy diet and kept on walking daily. After a year, she had lost 50 pounds and at two years she had attained a normal weight of 125 pounds. She felt great and looked great.

Ironically, her ex-husband and his new wife "found" the weight she lost. Now they are both overweight and uncomfortable.

11. DON'T BE AFRAID OF HUNGER.

Hunger is your friend. Hunger, while unpleasant, won't kill you. It's actually your body telling you, "Hey! We're losing weight right now!

Many of us eat by the clock. "It's noon, so it's time for lunch"; not "It's noon, and it's time for lunch, but I'm not that hungry at the moment, so I'm going to wait a while to eat." To make matters worse, we often stuff ourselves until we're full or even beyond, to the point of physical discomfort. We do this in part because it is our habit.

But it is also often in our genetics to over-eat. Your body wants you to live, and has a specific weight it wants you to maintain, give or take a few pounds. Scientists who study eating and obesity call this specific weight where you want to be your *set point*. Depending on your genetics, you may have either a higher or a lower set point.[19]

The set point is a big reason crash/starvation dieting so often fails. A person may change calorie intake, but the set point remains the same, and the body nags and nags through incessant hunger until the set point is once again met. In fact, our bodies revolt against starvation and actually drive us to overeat, to "overshoot" our set point. This fact has been known for some time. A study detailing this pitfall of rapid weight loss explains the aftermath of the classic semi-starvation study performed by nutritionist and weight loss pioneer Ansel Keys. (Keys also pioneered the Mediterranean diet and also lived to be 100 years old.) In his semi-starvation study, volunteers who went on a starvation diet lost 66 percent of their initial fat mass. After the study ended, the participants packed on the pounds. When they could eat whatever they chose, they regained their fat mass and much more, reaching 145 percent from where they began, far overshooting their respective set points. Subjects reported they felt like they could never get enough food.[20]

Theories on why we're driven to overcompensate after we drop below our set points suggest we are unconsciously preparing for future starvation, protecting ourselves with a layer of stored fat.

But all is not hopeless. Set points are *adjustable*. I call this the "floating" set point. Researchers David S. Ludwig and Mark I. Friedman wondered why obesity rates have increased three times as much since the 1960s when it is normal for the body to resist weight changes.

They found it is not overeating that is making us fatter, but the calories we lock away in fat tissue that is doing it. When we lock fat away, there is less available in the blood to satisfy the body's needs. We have a lot of calories in the wrong place. As a result, we get hungry because we are fatter.[21] In other words, when we gain weight, we tweak our set point. Upwards. One can easily see how weight-gain turns into a vicious cycle.

The Beth Israel Deaconess Medical Center, in conjunction with Harvard Medical School Teaching Hospital, has published "The Science of Set Point," which offers the most emphatic information I've seen for understanding and dealing with the Floating Set Point:

> Your heredity and your environment—starting back at the moment of your conception—determine your set point. Over the long term, excess food and insufficient exercise will override your body's natural tendency to stay at its set point and lead to a higher, less healthy set point. A slow, gradual weight gain will fool your body into thinking your set point should be higher—and in fact, that does reset your set point. Then, when you try to lose weight, your body defends that higher weight, making weight loss more difficult.[22]

But just as it's possible to reset your set point to a higher point, it's also possible to lower it. The secret is to work with, not against, your body's natural tendencies and lose weight *slowly*. Again, keep it to one pound a week. Understand at first, your body will resist this and attempt to keep you at your higher weight/set point. You may be very hungry at first. Don't be afraid of hunger; this is you beating and lowering your set point.

12. REMEMBER WHO'S IN CHARGE.

You are. You may feel out of control, like you just can't stop yourself. That's an illusion. No one can *make* you fail, and only you can make you succeed. Yes, you can. Yes, you *will*.

WHAT DAVE DOES

In the gym: four–six times per week (six is a good week):

Personal Maxim: Getting yourself to the gym is at least 50 percent of the workout.

Daily Gym Goal: Do your workout and leave uninjured.

Out of the gym:

Goal: at least 30 consistent minutes a day of some kind of physical activity such as walking, hiking, biking, swimming, and dancing.

WHAT ROBIN DOES

In the gym: I am not as fanatical about the gym as Dave. I go twice a week. I drag my butt in to work with a trainer for an hour each time. She has me doing weights on pulleys, kettlebells, squats with weights, and all kinds of things. I complain, but I have seen positive changes and I am strong because of my consistent visits.

Out of the gym: I hike five miles at least three days a week. In addition, I do Hip-Hop dancing for at least an hour a week and dance West Coast Swing two to three times a week. I also walk my demanding dog two to three times a day, rain or shine!

There are shortcuts to happiness,
and dancing is one of them.

—*VICKI BAUM*

PART IV
DANCE LIKE YOUR LIFE DEPENDS ON IT . . .

INTRODUCTION: ONE OF THE BEST THINGS YOU CAN DO

If we told you there is something available that would keep you young, fit, healthy, and bring you great balance and fun and it is practically free, would you be interested?

There is—that something is ballroom dance. Dance has been a part of rituals, celebration and healing—it has been an essential part of life—for eons. It is available to almost everyone, and for many it has become a true passion. What most people may not realize is dance, specifically ballroom dance, gives huge benefits beyond just enjoying a turn around the room.

Recent studies have found the key to happiness is love and connection.[1] That can be love of another person and/or of something that brings joy, such as music in the case of Beethoven, or dance, as in the case of the two of us—and that is why we knew we had to include it in this book!

Dance is great for overall health, in particular ballroom dance, with a growing body of scientific evidence to back up the emotional and physical benefits it brings. We will share these with you along with many stories of why it has become such a passion for an ever-growing number of people. We will start by explaining how and why we started dancing and why it has become such an important part of our lives and could become such an important part of yours.

DAVE KAHN'S STORY: A PATHWAY TO HAPPINESS

When I was a boy I had zero interest in dancing. My best bud (that would be Matt Murphy, mentioned earlier) and I were focused on turning over rocks and finding creepy-crawlies, riding our bikes, and target practice with our trusty BB guns. Dancing? For girls. The light wouldn't go on for years, not until I was an undergrad at UCLA. One day on my way to a workout at the John Wooden Center, I saw the "Learn to Dance!" flyer.

Mildly curious, I went. The class was packed, taught by a little old man with a bow tie and a checker coat, a stack of records under one arm, and under the other, an old-fashioned record player in a box. This was the time of DVDs, but he was clearly oblivious. He was awesome! In four weeks he had all of us doing the Foxtrot, Rumba, Waltz and Polka. I was hooked, and twenty-plus years later I still am.

The allure for me then was similar to what it is now. Happiness. That's the answer distilled into its simplest form. Today I walk into a dance full of people. They are usually all different ages, from every socioeconomic level. Not all of them are necessarily happy people, some perhaps may not be at all content in their lives, but for that moment they are coming together to find and create joy—immediate and shared gratification.

When I dance, I'm not only happy, I'm present. It's my habit to think ahead. Normally, thinking ahead is a good character trait; we thinkers are planners and we're prepared. But this takes us out of the moment, and while we busily ponder possible futures, we distract ourselves from marveling and indulging in the now. Dancing demands that one stays on time and in time and doesn't allow for wanderings. I find some of my very best moments are when I'm on the dance floor, balanced in the helix swirl and rhythm spin in the music, my partner and my self.

> *"There is an ecstasy that marks the summit of life, and beyond which life cannot rise. And such is the paradox of living, this ecstasy comes when one is most alive, and it comes as a complete forgetfulness that one is alive."*
>
> —Jack London, *The Call of the Wild*

ROBIN MILLER'S STORY: CONFESSIONS OF A KLUTZ

I started dancing when I was ten years old. My mother thought it would help me to be less of a klutz. She was worried about me; I had the uncanny ability of being able to fall off a chair spontaneously. I could also trip up any flight of stairs at a moment's notice. I started with ballet, and surprisingly when I focused on my steps, I could be quite graceful. So, I kept going with ballet and modern (now known as contemporary) dance. When I went away to college, my dance went by the wayside. I buried my nose in books and medical training and dance was a fond memory until . . .

About five years ago I was asked to participate in our local "Dancing with the Stars" competition to raise money for Sparrow Club, an organization which helps children fight diseases such as cancer and heart disease. I went to the first meeting for the competition and was introduced to various dances. They had semi-pro couples giving demonstrations. My eyes were drawn to one couple in particular. They were doing the Argentine tango. I took one look at the male lead dancer and said, "If I can dance with him,

I will do any dance you like!" And that was the beginning of my ballroom dance life.

Since I had such a great time and realized how wonderful ballroom dancing could be, after the competition I kept on dancing. That is when I met Dave. I started taking his West Coast Swing dance classes. He is a great instructor and an accomplished nationally competitive dancer. He got me to the point that I feel good about my dance—whether I am dancing with a novice or an advanced dancer. I love dancing so much, that I do it at least three times a week.

Why do I do it? There are so many reasons. One of the main reasons is because I have to focus on the dance in order to stay upright (I am still a klutz . . . we decided it is genetic), and all the thoughts and worries of my day have to melt away. For those three to four minutes, I am focused on one thing and one thing only, following my partner and maintaining the connection. In this crazy age where there are so many things bombarding us and draining our energy, it is so good to find something that requires me to be fully present in the moment.

Another great reason: my body got tighter! I noticed very soon after the competition I was building muscle and my clothes were fitting more loosely. I had to go out and buy a whole new wardrobe (a definite benefit!). My posture improved. As a result, my chronic neck pain, which had been there since I landed on my head in gymnastics class at the age of 12, was gone. I felt more awake and had more stamina, and mentally I felt sharper. Probably the most surprising thing is although I have always been a pretty happy person, since I have been dancing I have found an even greater level of happiness. I don't want to sound corny, but dancing brings me a level of joy that is indescribable.

As a doctor, I now regularly prescribe dancing to my patients. Every single one who has followed my prescription has found similar benefits. The beauty of ballroom dancing is you don't have to be a great dancer to get results. In addition, there are scientifically proven health benefits to dancing that will surprise you.

In this section of the book we will show you why it is important for you to get up and dance. There is good scientific evidence to show a variety of medical conditions can be improved with ballroom or partner dancing. Even if you are healthy, dance will allow you to maximize your health physically as well as emotionally.

Please join us as we make the case for why YOU should get up, find a partner and DANCE!

11 BRAIN POWER

AS I STATED IN Part I of this book, whenever I ask patients what their biggest fear is regarding their health, the answer is fairly unanimous. They are most afraid of losing their minds. If you gave people a choice between getting cancer or Alzheimer's, the majority would pick cancer.

THE STORY

Alfred was a 72-year-old gentleman who had lost his wife to ovarian cancer.

Soon after, his family became quite concerned about his memory. They noticed he was not as sharp as he had been, and he became confused easily. Sometimes he would get lost on his way home. Their concern was intensified due to the fact that he had a strong family history of Alzheimer's disease.

In an effort to soothe his loneliness, Alfred took up ballroom dancing, and things changed dramatically.

Soon after he started, his thinking became clearer and he was much happier.

At his favorite dance venue he met a lovely woman, and the two started dancing several times a week. He and his dancing friend have continued for over ten years. Alfred's mental function has remained intact; he has never developed any signs of dementia, and neither has his partner, who is well into her 90s.

Experts and Evidence

So far, there are no treatments available to halt or reverse Alzheimer's. So, what we must do is find ways to prevent it. There appear to be a few things that may have an impact. These are healthy eating, which we talked about in Part I, social engagement and exercise.

Exercise is clearly essential, and when it comes to Alzheimer's, there is an important extra element: social engagement. One of the most fascinating studies to date on this subject is the Nun Study. This is a longitudinal study that was started in 1986. Over 700 nuns and priests have had their mental and physical health followed throughout their lives—and beyond. Their activities, thoughts, and feelings are monitored and noted, and have been catalogued. They have yearly physical and cognitive exams. They have donated their bodies to science, and when they die their brains are analyzed.

Now beyond its 30th year, the study has found those who frequently participated in activities such as listening to the radio, reading newspapers, playing puzzle games and visiting museums were 47 percent less likely to develop Alzheimer's than those who did not. What is most intriguing about this study is there were 15 nuns who showed no signs of dementia in life, but when their brains were analyzed, they were diagnosed as having severe Alzheimer's. Their brains were loaded with the telltale plaque associated with the disease. When researchers looked back at their writing and activities, they found those women had a strong positive outlook and a sense of purpose in their lives. Being active is also important, and finding an activity that encourages social engagement is a win–win.[1]

Exercise is important for general health. Having a healthy heart and vascular system is important for having a healthy brain. The question is, which activities provide the *most* benefit? In 2003, a study published in the New England Journal of Medicine helped to answer that question. Researchers studied 469 people between the ages of 75 and 85. Participants answered surveys that addressed their activities such as walking, bicycling, reading, doing crossword puzzles and dancing. They were followed for five years. At the end of the study 124 had dementia.

Those who danced frequently had a lower risk of dementia when compared to those who did not dance. The risk of dementia was reduced by zero percent in those who were regular cyclists and swimmers, zero percent for the regular golfers, 35 percent reduced in those who were regular readers, 47 percent reduced by those who did crossword puzzles at least four times a week—and reduced by a stunning 76 percent for those who were partner dancing two to three times a week.[2]

Scientists have studied why dancing is so good for the brain. The cerebral cortex and the hippocampus parts of the brain are very plastic and can be easily rewired. That is a good thing. The downside is if you don't use them, you lose them. Partner dancing in particular requires multiple split–second decisions that are great for exercising the brain, and therefore keeps these essential parts of the brain highly functional.[3] As we age, creating more neural pathways in the brain improves brain function and gives us more reserve should there be an injury, and in the meantime, it keeps us mentally sharp.

One might look at the study above and wonder about the results since the activities were self-reported and it was an observational study rather than a true clinical trial. So you might ask the question:

has a clinical trial looking at subjects before and after dance training ever been done? And the answer is *yes*. The researchers looked at dancing the Cha-Cha and cognitive function in older subjects. A group of 38 seniors with metabolic syndrome (prediabetes) with normal cognitive function were divided into two groups. One group danced the Cha-Cha twice a week for six months. The other group followed their regular exercise routine. The dancing group showed improved cognition compared to the control group. The researchers came to the conclusion looking at verbal fluency, and word list recall and recognition after a time delay.

What sort of effect is seen in the brain with this type of activity? Radiologists at University of California Los Angeles were able to shed some light on this.[4] They studied 20 years of data from a group of 876 adults who averaged 78 years of age. This data looked at weight and height and lifestyle habits. They used special scans using magnetic resonance imaging (MRI) that established 3–D images of the brains of these individuals. With these, they were able to measure the amount of gray matter of the brain used for memory and decision-making. The more gray matter, the more brain power. This area shrinks in those with Alzheimer's disease. The researchers found those who were the most active had more gray matter than those who were not active. A combination of healthy lifestyle choices and activities was most beneficial. The researchers attributed these positive changes to improved blood flow to the brain and stronger neural connections.[5]

The bottom line is in order to keep from losing brain function, we need to harness our own brainpower. Embracing a healthy lifestyle with a whole food, Mediterranean-style diet, social interaction and exercise can do it. However, not just any exercise will do when it comes to growing neural connections and protecting the brain from Alzheimer's disease. Crossword puzzles and reading can help for brain exercise. However, for the most beneficial and expeditious results, ballroom dancing is the best choice. It exercises the body as well as the mind and is fun. It also provides many other benefits, as you will soon see.

PARKINSON'S DISEASE AND DANCE:
HOW TO STOP SHAKING, RATTLING AND ROLLING!

Even if you haven't had direct experience with Parkinson's disease, you may be aware of the disease because of the actor Michael J. Fox. By his choice to stay in the public eye and his continuing to work while he struggles with the disease, we have all become familiar with what it does.

THE STORY

Carlos is a 61-year-old accomplished ballroom dancer who had been dancing Salsa for years. He started noticing hand and arm tremors at the age of 47 and was diagnosed with Parkinson's disease seven years later. Parkinson's disease makes movement difficult and requires the need to be conscious of every step. For Carlos walking is a chore. Eight years ago, he started dancing the Argentine tango. He noticed it made his movement easier. He has realized Parkinson's disease keeps his weight over his heels, and Tango helps to keep his body forward and improves his backward stride and balance.

Tango keeps Carlos moving. Every morning, he watches his favorite Tango dancer on YouTube. Inspired by this man, he puts on his Tango music and practices his stride. He credits Tango and dance with the ability to ride his bike and walk to wherever he needs to go. His dance instructor finds that when Carlos dances, his whole body relaxes into the dance and his tremors decrease. Carlos's goal is to retire early so he can have more fun and dance more often.

Experts and Evidence

Parkinson's disease is a progressive disease of the nervous system. For a detailed description of Parkinson's causes and symptoms see Chapter 4. In essence, patients have a deficiency of a chemical transmitted by the nervous system called dopamine. As a result, patients develop tremors, rigid muscles, and have very poor balance with the tendency to fall forward. Some patients' experience "freezing," which is the temporary, involuntary inability to move. This increases the likelihood of falling. It can be extremely dangerous.

Therapy focuses on exercise and stretching. This is tough for many patients to do on a consistent basis. However, there is a form of physical activity that helps and patients actually *like* to do. This activity is ballroom dancing; more specifically Tango.[6]

Dr. Gammon Earhart, an esteemed Parkinson's researcher and her team did a recent study at Washington University, St. Louis. They took 52 patients with Parkinson's disease who had similar problems with movement and balance. Half the group was given Tango lessons twice weekly for a year, and the other half maintained their normal activity level. Improvement in symptoms of Parkinson's disease was noted in many of the Tango students. They were able to walk faster and farther, and their balance improved. The non-Tango group either remained unchanged or worsened over the year. Those who did the Tango also were more active in their lives. They became more social, did more daily activities at home, such as gardening and shopping, and enjoyed going to movies and eating out. These improvements diminished when they stopped dancing. However, most people in the study enjoyed doing Tango and continued to dance.[7]

You may be asking, why *Tango*? These same researchers looked at the effects of other forms of ballroom dancing on movement and balance for Parkinson's disease patients.

In another study, 58 untreated patients with Parkinson's disease were randomly assigned to one of three groups, a control group with no intervention, a Waltz/Foxtrot group or a Tango group. They had 20 training sessions over a 13–week period.

Both dance groups improved with respect to balance, motor ability and walking. The control group worsened by 24 percent on scales that rate the above factors. Tango was superior to Waltz and Foxtrot when it came to freezing movements in Parkinson's disease. In addition, the speed and stride length of walking improved more with Tango.[8]

What is it about dance and specifically Tango that may be helping? First of all, dancing offers external cues for movement from the music and a partner. These cues bypass the part of the brain that is dysfunctional. This in turn improves gait and coordination. Touch from a partner improves balance. In Tango, visual clues that involve stepping over a partner's foot or crossing one foot over another help prevent the serious symptom of Parkinson's known as freezing of the gait. The need for forward and backward steps in Tango is particularly therapeutic for those with Parkinson's disease.

There is a special radiologic imaging test called a PET (positron emission tomography) scan that shows brain activity in real time. A PET scan was done of Tango dancers and showed increased activity in the part of the brain that is dysfunctional in Parkinson's disease patients when tango movements were done to a regular, predictable beat.

It is tough for many of us to get motivated to exercise. For Parkinson's disease patients who suffer from muscle pain and rigidity, loss of balance and generalized stiffness, it is even harder. Tango offers pain relief, improvement in balance and a better quality of life. The best part is it is fun and very inexpensive. All you need is a decent pair of shoes and a Tango class. You also may want to explore the website danceforparkinsons.org. It offers extensive information and opportunities to explore dance as a viable therapy for patients with Parkinson's disease.

TBI: DANCE AWAY THE TRAUMA

There is very little research on the use of dance for traumatic brain injury. What has been studied is the helpful effect of rhythmic movement and the resulting improvement in patients with TBI.

THE STORY
John is the 19-year-old competitive dancer I mentioned previously who had been in a horrific car accident. He was in a coma and suffered serious head trauma. His speech and

thinking were slowed, he had left-sided weakness, and his doctors and therapists doubted he would ever walk normally, much less dance. However, after three months he was back doing West Coast Swing. He persevered, and along with his athletic abilities, his speech and thinking improved. Three years later, he is better than ever. He attributes his work and love of dance to his remarkable improvement. When asked what dance means to him, he smiles, "Dance is my passion, my motivation, my future."

Experts and Evidence

There is one small, landmark study looking at movement and improvement with TBI. Dr. Corene Hurt studied eight patients post-injury. She and her group measured their ability to walk symmetrically and to walk to the rhythm of the music. They also measured their speed of walking. After training to music daily for five weeks, five of the patients improved significantly.[9]

Researchers are now looking at using dance to help improve TBI, since through studies of other neurologic conditions we know it can improve physical and cognitive function. The key is to find a therapy that works and helps patients to stay with it.

Getting patients to go to physical therapy and rehab on a regular basis is often challenging. Having an activity they enjoy is a great motivator to help them heal their brains. There are many studies showing the enjoyment factor of exercise influences long-term participation.[10]

12 Finally! A Program Just For You

WATCHING COMPETITIVE DANCING is fun for most of us. It is inspiring as well as entertaining.

> **THE STORY**
>
> If you are a fan of the ABC show Dancing with the Stars, then you have watched some amazing transformations, and I am not just talking about the dancing. I am referring to the body changes that occur in many of the stars who start out overweight and slim down to a healthy weight. Granted, the show has grueling rehearsals and makes it a lot easier for weight loss to happen. However, these people show us how fun and effective dance can be for weight loss.
>
> The first winner of Dancing with the Stars was John O'Hurley. He was not obese at the outset, but he was out of shape. As the competition progressed, he experienced a healthy weight loss that resulted in improved energy and enthusiasm.

> Others have thinned down remarkably before our eyes. Kirstie Alley lost 20 pounds, Kelly Osbourne lost 42 pounds, Jane Seymour lost 22 pounds, Marie Osmond 31 pounds, Lil' Kim 20 pounds, Kyle Massie 18 pounds and Gladys Knight lost a whopping 60 pounds!

WEIGHT LOSS DOES NOT HAVE TO EQUAL MISERY

A study published in the Journal of the American Medical Association found exercise alone does not result in weight loss. It needs to be coupled with a healthy diet. That being said, if you want to lose weight, exercise is important to burn the healthy calories you do consume.[1]

Unfortunately, many people hate to exercise. In fact, studies done by the CDC have shown only 30 percent of Americans report they exercise regularly, and 40 percent say they do not exercise at all. What is really scary is studies that measure actual physical activity using motion detectors find people overestimate how much exercise they actually perform.[2]

That is why it is important to find something fun you like to do which coincidentally happens to burn calories. *Dancing is that activity.* It is fun and it does help with weight loss among many other benefits.

> A study took 60 Japanese women who were overweight, and over three months they participated in a weight loss program that encompassed diet and exercise. The subjects were divided into two groups: they either did aerobic dance or they did jogging and/or cycling. Both groups lost around seven pounds and about six percent body fat. Both forms of exercise worked. This study illustrates, at minimum, dance is comparable to more traditional forms of exercise.[3]

Now let's talk long-term. In 2012, a study of 100 overweight individuals between the ages of 40 and 70 were either given two-hour dance sessions with Latin and Standard Ballroom dancing twice weekly for six months or a self-selected sports activity that could include cycling, aerobics, walking or swimming. At three months, both groups had lost an average of about six pounds and had taken about 1.5 inches off their waistlines. This was maintained at six months. However, only the dance group was able to keep up the same high activity level after six months; the dropout rate was much higher for the exercise group. That is because the dancers enjoyed themselves, so they kept on dancing.[4]

Dance is fun and as a result the benefits of weight loss and fitness have not been lost on the public. In fact, dance is the fastest growing exercise and art form in Britain. More than 4.8 million people regularly attend community dance groups there each year.[5]

How many calories are they burning while enjoying themselves? Slow ballroom dancing burns 207 calories an hour, and fast ballroom dancing can burn as many as 378 calories an hour. Swing burns 306 an hour and hip-hop burns the most at 465 calories an hour.[6]

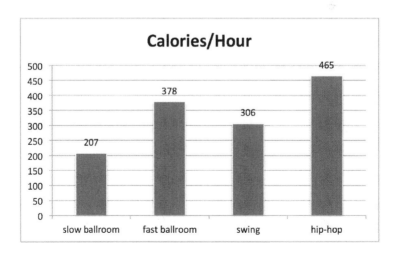

DANCE DIABETES AWAY

In addition to helping overweight people to lose weight, dancing also helps to treat and prevent type 2 diabetes, a disease which often occurs as a result of obesity. Read on.

> **THE STORY**
>
> Joseph is a 65-year-old-man who has had type 2 diabetes for ten years. He took medication and maintained a normal blood sugar, but he never felt good. He was overweight and finally decided it was time to change. He had always enjoyed ballroom dancing, and therefore he increased the hours he danced each week, changed his diet to whole foods, and he cut out the junk food. He lost 40 pounds in a matter of months, stopped his medication and is feeling better than he has in years.

Experts and Evidence

We know the prevention and treatment of type 2 diabetes includes healthy whole foods, a low carbohydrate diet, and exercise. The problem is many diabetics do not like to exercise. In fact, a review of a large population survey found diabetics exercise less than those without diabetes. The most common activity they were engaged in was walking. They were less likely to jog, dance, cycle, lift weights, and ski when compared to those who did not have diabetes.[7]

In the 2012 study of exercise and obesity mentioned earlier in this chapter, those with diabetes were studied as well. Comparing those who did Latin and Standard Ballroom dancing to those who did regular exercise, at six months the dancing group had maintained a lower hemoglobin A1C level, reflecting better diabetes control as compared to those in the regular exercise program. Dancing is an effective activity for control of blood sugar.

The general recommendations for exercise for diabetics include:

➥ Doing aerobic activity at least 30 minutes a day, four or more days a week.

➥ Work up to your maintenance level of exercise gradually if you have not exercised regularly.

➥ Find an exercise that you like so you will keep doing it.

➥ Schedule your exercise at the same time each day to help with blood sugar control.

Dancing can easily fit all these recommendations!

An organization called T2 Dance Crew, set up by Debbie Allen, the award winning actress, dancer and choreographer, encourages those with type 2 diabetes to get moving and enjoy dance as a fun, sustainable, healthy activity. The organization has a video that helps those with type 2 diabetes get started slowly. T2 Dance Crew shares a wide variety of dances, they host events that teach dance classes live via video link, and they provide health screenings around the country. Their website is T2DanceCrew.com.

Dance can help fight obesity among a variety of health problems. Whether you are overweight or you are pre-diabetic, diabetic or just looking to stay at a healthy weight, it is time to get out there and dance!

13 LOWER YOUR BLOOD PRESSURE

ONE OF THE most common pieces of advice for people with high blood pressure or other risk factors for heart disease such as high cholesterol, obesity and sedentary behavior is to exercise. Yet, few patients actually follow this advice. The problem is that it is really hard to get people to do it.

THE STORY

Phil is a 60-year-old Filipino man who was diagnosed with high blood pressure and was on medication. Five years ago, he started partner dancing. His doctor noted each year his blood pressure was lower than the year before, until finally his blood pressure medication was completely discontinued. His weight has decreased along with his blood pressure, and to this day he is feeling fantastic.

Experts and Evidence

Since exercise is so important for high blood pressure control, there have been several studies conducted to see if there is something fun and entertaining enough to get people moving and keep them moving.

A recent study conducted by the Centers for Disease Control found nearly 80 percent of Americans do not get their recommended amount of exercise. Researchers surveyed 450,000 adults in the United States over the age of 18. About 23 percent of all the men and 18 percent of the women met the recommended exercise requirements. People between 18 and 24 were most likely to exercise and those over 65 were least likely to exercise.[1]

Scientists have looked at what motivates us to move. From studies on identical twins, it has been verified there is a genetic component that regulates our exercise. When twins have grown up in different environments, they still have similar exercise habits.[2] Further studies have found those who have fun exercising are more likely to engage in it.[3] The key is to find a way for it to be enjoyable.

> A study followed 37 Filipino Americans between the age of 35 and 65 who entered into a ballroom dance program. They were taught Cha-Cha, Rumba and Salsa every week for two hours over three months. At the end of the study period, their blood pressure, heart rates, weight, and waist circumference were all reduced. At the end of the study, the majority of the dancers were still dancing and enjoying it.[4]
>
> A study that looked specifically at those on medication for blood pressure has found similar results.[4] Twenty-three patients who averaged 62 years of age danced three times a week for 40 one-hour sessions. The dances consisted of Bolero, Brazillian Rock ,Forro, Merengue, Salsa, and Samba. Blood pressure was checked after each session. When compared to walking and a mixed exercise program, dancing showed the best results at lowering systolic (the upper) blood pressure.

The lowering of diastolic blood pressure was similar in all types of exercise. The blood pressure reduction was maintained for at least 48 hours. If patients dance three days a week, they can maintain lower pressures indefinitely.

In general, 40 percent of people will stick with a walking program. After the three-month dance program, 90 percent were still dancing.

Finally, a study of 110 heart failure patients found dancing the Waltz three times a week for eight weeks was equally as effective at improving heart function as walking on a treadmill or cycling. The biggest difference between these different exercise groups is the dancers experienced an improved quality of life when compared to the other groups—and no one was injured! [5]

Ballroom dancing is relatively safe and very effective when it comes to improving cardiovascular health. In addition, because it is so much fun and helps people to feel better immediately, they want to keep doing it.

14 Finding the Right Balance—Literally

AS WE AGE, balance and the chance of falling become more of an issue for our general health and well being. Just one major fall can be devastating

> **DAVE'S STORY**
>
> I loved my grandmother, Blanche Kahn, very much. She lived long enough and stayed present long enough, both mentally and physically, to become more to me than the typical grandmother; as I grew into adulthood, we became dear friends. We'd get together at least once a week and often talk in between. I was a young man then, but old enough to truly understand the treasure of the relationship.
>
> Because we were so close, I could talk to Blanche frankly about her health and her weight. Her choices weren't good ones. She was never one for doing much in way of exercise or healthy eating, and like many of her generation, she smoked for the majority of her life. Living in a health-conscious way just wasn't a priority for her. I'd remind

and cajole, but stopped short of nagging. Blanche made it clear she wasn't going to change, so there was no point in badgering her. She was the way she was, she explained, and she truly believed it was too late for her to do things differently.

As Blanche got older, she grew more frail. In part because of the way she lived her life, she eventually got very sick. She had to face a major operation and a major recovery, but she was strong and she was a fighter. As she struggled to recover, it was the falls that were hindering her. That time was scary for all of us, especially for Blanche. She grew terrified of another setback, but try as she might, she simply couldn't keep her balance. After her third major fall, she was readmitted to the hospital, and she died soon after. It's been more than 15 years, and I still poignantly miss her.

Experts and Evidence

The statistics are daunting. The Centers for Disease Control point out just how common it is for older people (65+) to suffer from falling: "Each year, 2.5 million older people are treated in emergency departments for fall injuries" with often life-changing consequence. "Among older adults, falls are the number one cause of fractures, hospital admissions for trauma, loss of independence, and injury deaths."[1] Furthermore, falling once doubles your chances of falling again; a serious fall is rarely just a one–time event.[2]

Why are serious falls such a common phenomenon, especially for older adults? There are a number of risk factors ranging from poor reactions to certain medications to a lack of vitamin D. However, two of the biggest contributing factors are lack of muscle strength and a decline in balance.[3] These two major issues are compounded as we age. There have been many studies that show a decline in strength, motor skills, balance and our ability to react to different stimuli as we become older.

However, it's not all bad news. Studies have also found this decline is variable and depends on one's proficiency at different activities. In fact, some older individuals lose little to any skill as they age. You can see this with professional musicians such as the Rolling Stones, BB King, and Itzhak Perlman; and also in athletes from diverse sports such as golf and bowling—even powerlifters can continue to lift much heavier-than-average-weight well into their 60s, 70s and even 80s.[4]

Nobody wants to fall and have to suffer the potentially horrific consequences. While there are many ways to stay in shape and reduce risk, there is no doubt having good balance strength is imperative. Knowing this, we know it is possible for older individuals to maintain and even improve their balance!

We also know of the many ways to achieve positive results in balance, ballroom dancing is one of the most effective. The data bears this out.

A study done in Germany evaluated 62 healthy, elderly volunteers living independently between the ages of 61 and 94. For the study they recruited two groups: one who had been long-time amateur dancers, 16.5 years on average, and another group who had never danced. Several measures were used to test each group's posture and balance. Not surprisingly, the dancer group was far superior to the non-dancer group on all of these measures.[5]

Those results were in people living independently. Would ballroom dance help those in assisted living to improve their posture and balance? Yes.

Researchers looked at 59 residents of a nursing home. Half were assigned to the ballroom dance group. They danced for 30 minutes three times a week for three months, while the other half were controls who were asked not to exercise for the study period (but were promised they could join the dance group when the study was finished).

The groups were tested for balance and the number of falls they had experienced in the prior three months. For 12 weeks, the dancers participated in dancing sessions that started with a ten–minute warm up session followed by 30 minutes of the Foxtrot, Waltz, Rumba, Swing, Samba or Bolero. Each session ended with a 10–minute relaxation period.

At the end of the study period, the dance group showed a 50 percent improvement in balance and a marked reduction in falls. The dancers also lost a significant amount of weight when compared to the control group. Predictably, the control group enthusiastically joined the dancers at the end of the study.[6] It's been literally proven: Ballroom dancing is a safe activity that improves balance in the elderly and reduces falls.

Knowing how effective ballroom dancing is for people in a nursing home, you might wonder how well professional dancers do as they age. Do they have even better balance and better physical performance overall?

Another study done in Germany addressed that question. They studied 49 healthy subjects. Eleven were competitive dancers. They were all on average 70 years of age. The study found the dancers performed better when it came to balance, posture and reaction times compared to the healthy control group that did not dance.[7]

This is good news for all of us who are amateurs. It appears the act of learning and becoming a dancer (good, bad or mediocre) is what provides the benefits.

We not only have the evidence from the studies; we have experienced the benefits of balance from ballroom dance firsthand:

ROBIN'S STORY

As I mentioned in the introduction of this book, I have always been a klutz. I used to trip and fall quite a bit. When I started ballroom dancing, I noticed my balance was pretty terrible. I would tilt when I turned and I felt off kilter.

In the beginning, I could do one or two turns and feel okay. Any more than that and I would feel nauseated and unsteady. I used to come home from my lessons and throw up (something I am sharing here for the first time). However, the more I danced, the less off balance I started to feel.

I am proud to share that now it no longer happens. I do not dread turning—now I actually enjoy it. I rarely trip when I am walking or climbing and descending stairs. I have excellent posture and I feel very confident in my stance.

My dancing has helped improve my balance, posture and agility!

15 Osteoporosis

OSTEOPOROSIS IS A widespread problem, affecting people the world over. According to the international osteoporosis foundation, it is responsible for more than 8.9 million fractures annually worldwide, which means an osteoporotic fracture occurs every three seconds. These occur in the hip, forearm and back. Those with a fractured hip or spine have an increased early mortality of ten percent to 20 percent. Fractures make moving around difficult, cause chronic pain and are often responsible for a loss of independence.[1, 2]

> **THE STORY**
>
> Jan is a 70-year-old woman who has an established family history of osteoporosis. She came to see me for a second opinion regarding her low bone density. She was diagnosed to be in an early stage of osteoporosis and was prescribed medication. She was very reluctant to take it. We agreed to try other measures first to see if we could improve her bones.

She started on vitamin D, dietary calcium and a special exercise program. She lifted weights two days a week with a trainer and started dancing three days a week. After a year, I rechecked her bone density, and she had no evidence of osteoporosis and very minimal early bone loss.

After three years, her bone density is now completely normal. In addition, with weight loss due to exercise, she has attained her ideal body weight and feels great.

Experts and Evidence

Osteoporosis occurs when we lose bone mass and density as we age. While men suffer from osteoporosis, post-menopausal women are at highest risk for bone loss since bone building is related to estrogen levels.

In addition to menopause, certain medications can increase the risk for osteoporosis. These include:

- Aluminum containing antacids
- Certain chemotherapy drugs
- Anti-seizure medication such as Dilantin
- Heparin
- Lithium
- Methotrexate
- Proton pump inhibitors such as Prilosec and Nexium
- Antidepressants such as Lexapro, Prozac and Zoloft
- Prednisone
- Tamoxifen

A family history of osteoporosis, cigarette smoking, excessive alcohol intake, lack of vitamin D and calcium in the diet, and a sedentary lifestyle all contribute to the risk of bone loss.

Treatment for osteoporosis includes lifestyle modification, dietary changes and may involve medication as well. Exercise is also very important, but not just any exercise. The type of exercise that reverses osteoporosis is that which pounds or stresses bones. Bones actually respond to weight bearing exercise by becoming denser and stronger. So, walking and weight (or resistance) training are key. Both the Surgeon General of the United States and the National Osteoporosis Foundation realize how important this is, and they recommend ballroom dancing as a form of exercise to treat and prevent osteoporosis.[3]

When patients have been diagnosed with osteoporosis, they generally know what they need to do to improve their bones. They have been told they need to have a regular exercise regimen. Unfortunately, approximately 24 percent of Americans have little or no physical activity in their daily lives, and only 49 percent do at least 30 minutes of moderate activity five or more days per week.[4] Again, success is challenged by this persistent problem: many people simply do not like to exercise and therefore they don't do it. Dancing is a great form of exercise because large muscle groups are utilized over relatively long periods of time. The mechanical weight bearing that occurs as a result improves bone density. Again, dancing is the answer, and because it's more fun and more social than most other forms of traditional exercise, people tend to stay with it.

16 DANCE FOR RECOVERY

SPEEDING YOUR RECOVERY FROM CANCER

Exercise is something typically recommended during and after patients have been treated for cancer. As we will note, multiple studies done on those with breast, colorectal, prostate and ovarian cancer have found patients who are physically active have a lower risk of the cancer returning and improved survival when compared to those who are inactive.[1]

> **THE STORY**
>
> Lisa is a 60-year-old woman who was diagnosed with both melanoma and breast cancer many years ago. She went for an unconventional treatment in Mexico and was cancer free until a couple of years ago when her breast cancer recurred.
>
> Lisa had been healthy until a series of very stressful life events took their toll. She lost her father and was divorced around the same time. Her husband of 24 years had been a

normal, reasonable man until he got into drugs. He became abusive and violent. She was forced to run from him with her children. He followed and had even kidnapped her children at one point. Fortunately, she was able to make it to her current location, and he is no longer a threat to her safety.

When her daughter was in high school, Lisa used to take her to ballroom dancing and wait in the car for her. However, when her daughter left to go to college, she decided to start dancing herself. She began with country dancing and progressed to ballroom dancing (Waltz, Cha Cha and Foxtrot) and has added West Coast Swing to her repertoire.

She credits dance for saving her life. Dance takes her pain away. It has also provided her with a social network and the solid support of close friends. She is getting a great deal of exercise because she dances anywhere from three to six days a week.

For Lisa, dance is her life and dance is freedom.

Experts and Evidence

A pilot study done at two cancer centers in Connecticut looked at the effect of dance and movement on the quality of life and shoulder function of breast cancer survivors treated within five years of diagnosis. A total of 35 women were studied over a 12–week period. The Lebed Method, Focus on Healing Through Movement and Dance, was used. This is a series of exercises that are simple and designed to improve the movement of lymph. There are simple dance movements taught as well.

One group received the treatment and the control group did not. After 12 weeks, the control group became the active group and the active group became the control group. Shoulder range of motion, body image and quality of life were studied at 12 and 24 weeks. Significant improvement was noted in all of the above factors.[2]

Unfortunately, there are no studies thus far that have looked specifically at ballroom dance and how it affects cancer patients. However, there are many people who use dancing to successfully cope with their recovery from cancer. A great example is Anada Shankar Jayant who has a TED talk describing how dance has been essential to her survival and recovery.

Can dance cure cancer? No, but it can make treatment and recovery a whole lot easier.

17 Social Anxiety? Not Any More!

CONSIDER THE LAST wedding reception you attended. When it was time for the guests to dance, you at first likely saw only a few step out onto the floor (the brave, the crazies and the drunks). After a while, some others were coaxed and cajoled and eventually got their courage up and reluctantly started to dance, while others refused to be dragged out under any circumstances—or they simply hid in the corner or up and left when the dancing started.

As rocker Morrissey of The Smiths wrote, *"Shyness can stop you from doing all the things in life you'd like to."* Social Anxiety, recognized by the medical community as an actual psychological disorder, goes much further; it can be utterly debilitating.

No matter where one may be placed on the spectrum, from a case of shyness to true social anxiety (SA), the mere idea of dancing strikes fear into the hearts (and feet) of many.

What's this about? Why are some people so averse to dancing? Insecurity. No one ever wants to feel awkward or stupid, or to be laughed at. Some people go their whole lives avoiding dancing; if they must dance, it's only when forced and/or inebriated.

For others, the social anxiety they feel on a day-to-day basis not only puts dancing completely out of the question, it makes most social situations stressful. Parties, groups of people, public gatherings or celebrations are not things to be enjoyed, but endured or (preferably) avoided entirely.

THE STORIES

UCHIKI

Uchiki was a very shy, reserved girl by nature. In addition, she was raised with a traditional Japanese ethos, which meant any kind of extroversion was frowned upon. In America as a grown woman, she was still always the quiet one, and although she couldn't admit it to herself at the time, she lived her life walled off from being how she truly wanted to be, from being her true self. For Uchiki, dancing changed everything.

One day, a friend saw her moving to a song at a party and asked her to come to a dance lesson with her. After weeks of relentless prodding, she went reluctantly. She was surprised to find she really liked it. And she realized an added benefit: she could be social without having to talk to anyone.

Initially, the toughest part of dancing for Uchiki was touching a man's hand and making eye contact. The more she danced, the easier it was to get over that hurdle. She realizes dancing has made her feel free to be who she truly is. Her life had always consisted of caring for her grandmother and mother, and then her husband and son. However, her marriage ended (amicably) and her son grew up and left home. She found herself with some new and unfamiliar freedom and the opportunity arose for her to enjoy it. Dancing is still with her and has given her a new life. It has opened her up to an entire group of friends and dance partners. She has come out of her shell and can make eye contact—and even on occasion flirt a bit.

For Uchiki, dance is love, joy and gratitude.

DINA

Dina is a woman in her early twenties who started dancing as a young girl. As a child, she was plagued with shyness. Dancing has helped her to get out of her shell and to be more outgoing. She is now a West Coast Swing champion. She has become a teacher of dance and travels all over the world competing. This skill has translated into more confidence in her working life. Her desire for excellence in dance has also inspired her to eat healthy and be active. She found a healthy lifestyle helped her dance, and she felt better overall. Dancing has enhanced her sense of well being and brings her joy and happiness. It has also brought her a boyfriend who feels similarly about dance.

MARK

Mark is a professional West Coast Swing dancer. He started dancing about ten years ago while in college. He was looking for a fun form of physical activity, and his girlfriend at the time suggested they try dancing. He tried it and did like it, but life intervened and he had to leave it, along with college. When he returned to college a couple of years later (and single), he decided to try it again. He took a dance class and hated it. He was about to drop the class, but at the moment before hitting the "withdraw" button on the computer, he hesitated. He examined his motivation to quit: ballroom dance made him uncomfortable. He would have to interact with people he did not know, and he would have to show himself in a way he sometimes did not like; he felt vulnerable. That realization encouraged him to make the decision to stay and to use it as a challenge and an opportunity to grow. He didn't hit that button. Instead, he kept working at dance and found he really started to like it. Shortly thereafter, he was hooked. It led to his present career as a dance teacher and also his romantic relationship with a fellow dancer.

For Mark, dancing means growth and pushing himself. He gets a lot of satisfaction from it. Being able to interact with many people is now appealing to him. And he enjoys the technique part, too; that includes the challenge of working on something until he gets it, to doing it until he gets it right, and then knowing he has it. He can see the results, in himself, but especially in the people he is dancing with. They dance better because he's dancing better.

The other thing that has happened for him recently, especially as he has become better in his own movement, is the expression to the music has become much more important. Now that he has that skill, dancing has become even more enjoyable. He has found a new way to enjoy dancing simply because his skill level has increased. Had he not pushed himself, he never would have found it. Had he not grown in that direction, beyond feeling uncomfortable, he would have missed all the enjoyment and the empowering sense of well-being.

Experts and Evidence

You don't have to be diagnosed with a full-blown case of social anxiety to benefit from the strategies and treatments used for dealing with it. According to the experts, shyness and SA are part of the same continuum. Social anxiety is simply more severe. So even if you struggle just occasionally with shyness or self-esteem, you can be helped.

With the above in mind, there is a lot of evidence that confirms SA is successfully treated through dance. Dr. Thomas A. Richards, Ph.D., psychologist and founder of the Social Anxiety Institute, talks about the importance of using Cognitive–Behavioral Therapy (CBT) to treat SA. A big part of the therapy is being proactive; it is important to take the initiative when things happen in life rather than just responding when things happen to you.

"Dance lessons are a way to be proactive by working on self-consciousness. They help by making shy and/or anxious people talk with their dance partners. They also help students to learn to relax as much as possible, and focus on the instructions and moves being taught. In general these are effective strategies to put into place. Dancing is a great social activity to help with feeling comfortable in a safe environment." [1]

Dr. Bill Knaus wrote *the* book on overcoming social anxiety, *The Cognitive Behavioral Workbook for Anxiety*, as well as over 20 other books based on his experience as a clinical psychologist and former psychology professor. He describes a dance activity he led in a recent shyness and social anxiety workshop:

Immediately after the members introduced themselves and said what they'd like to get out of the workshop, he started a "Shy Away" dance exercise. The instructions: Pantomime shyness through dancing and gestures. Symbolically show what it is like to be shy. He started the dance. Within seconds, the entire group was doing the Shy Away.

He ended the exercise and then talked about whether anyone would ever consider doing a solo dance at a party. No one would. Some said if they had enough time to think about it, they might have bolted for the door.

What did each learn from the experience? He heard many perspectives. Some were amazed they could do it. Many realized how much fun they had when they loosened up and danced. Even those who were most anxious said it wasn't too bad. A few said the exercise was too easy. Most felt neither judged nor threatened. The Shy Away was a breakthrough exercise. [2]

In fact, there is an entire field of academic study and treatment devoted to healing through dance: Dance Movement Therapy. The American Dance Movement Therapy (ADMT) Association defines dance/movement therapy as the use of movement to further the emotional, cognitive, physical and social integration of the individual. It is effective for people with social, physical and psychological problems.[3]

Although the ADMT doesn't use specific forms of established partner dancing, their treatments tie in with what experts in partner dancing have learned from their students regarding anxiety:

"To see someone dance is to witness release, self-expression, and often joy. For many of those reasons, many therapists who treat anxiety are finding that dance has the potential to act as an effective treatment for anxiety." [4]

Dance Pizazz, a long-established dance studio in St. Louis, Missouri; puts a great spin on the social aspect of dance:

➥ Ballroom dancing is an excellent form of exercise— and fun! It is a workout for the mind and the body. It engages our cognitive and spatial ability: both key components in developing a stronger social skill-set. Therefore, the more the dancer dances, the less anxious and more social he/she can become thanks to this workout.

➥ Dancing, especially without a constant partner, leads to increased confidence. Dancers learn with and through others in a safe and relaxed environment.

➥ Because practice makes perfect, both private and group lessons present great opportunities for a dancer of any level to improve their craft through repetition. It's a fact: feeling more confident in any activity can considerably reduce anxiety.

➥ Social dancing improves communication. Anyone attending a group lesson already has at least one thing in common: they are interested in ballroom dance.

This presents a perfect icebreaker for safe mingling. Just having a basic conversation about the shared joys of dance can help anyone with their communication skills and, eventually, with their overall social competence.[5]

It may seem counter-intuitive, but the scariest of all possible social situations—dancing in public—is actually the key to feeling more confident and less awkward not only in dance, but in all social situations.

18 BREAKING GOOD

IN OUR PREVIOUS chapter, we discuss how dancing helps with
shyness and Social Anxiety, that is, how we feel about our interaction
with the outside world. Dancing helps as well with the way we feel
about our internal world: our self confidence.

THE STORY:

At the time we interviewed him, Jonathan appeared to us
as one of the happiest, and by far the most confident, of
the people we'd met during the writing of this book. At
first glance, one may be tempted to question why. While
he presents as kind and intelligent, he is not extravagantly
wealthy or overly-accomplished. While he is of average
complexion, he is clearly overweight and he is losing his
hair. But he has an easy, self-possessed way about him, and
a smile and a nod (or sometimes a shrug) that suggests he's
got things not only figured out, but he's got them going on.

We talked to Jonathan about dance, and it became clear for him, dancing was the key to his sense of well-being and his above-average composure. Talking to him, one would have no idea he'd ever been reserved or lacked confidence. "I needed to come out of my shell," he assured us.

Coming back from a stint in the military, he started to dance because he wanted to make friends and meet women, but also because he wanted to help—there was a shortage of leads in the local dance community. "I'd always had an attitude of serving, but I think this was a crutch to help with my low self-esteem. It allowed me to assume a role which helped me get past my hesitation." So he began taking lessons and playing the role, "serving a purpose," by making himself available to help out.

Not long into this new endeavor, he noticed a shift beginning within him. "Soon after I started dancing, my personality started to break through; dancing went from something I wanted to do because I was serving, to something I wanted to do because I truly liked it. And now because of dancing, I just don't hide from the world any more."

But this new-found benefit wasn't limited to the dance floor. "The confidence I found though dance got me to come out of hiding, and that same confidence transferred to the rest of my life." He started approaching relationships with women in an entirely different way. He explained that he used to feel like he had to constantly please the woman he was dating—with that same anxiety to serve. He was able to see such an approach not only wasn't what he wanted, but also such a disposition put him in a place of servility and weakness few women were drawn to.

Dancing taught him relationships on the dance floor are similar to those is life: sometimes they work and there will always be another dance as soon as you are ready. Just being his relaxed and newly-confident self started to work well for him. "I just stopped worrying about trying to hide myself in the role of server, something I had been doing for so terribly long; that's what dance has done for me."

Clearly, it's done quite a lot. And more. Since we spoke with him, Jonathan has gotten married—to one of his dance partners.

Experts and Evidence

Dr. Mark R. Leary, a Professor of Psychology at Duke University best describes Jonathan's experience in his paper, "The Interpersonal Basis of Self-Esteem." He concludes "believing that one possesses attributes that lead one to be valued by others will result in higher self-esteem." [1] This is what slowly happened to Jonathan. He started believing in himself, that he had value beyond that of simply being a pleaser, and he became more self confident.

However, for many there is a catch–22 regarding a lack of confidence and starting to dance: sure, dancing builds confidence, but if one needs confidence to get started dancing in order to build confidence, how can that possibly work? According to Dr. Leary, self-confidence is an important ingredient for success. If you don't have it, it is possible to *pretend* you do have it. Putting on a confident face will allow a person to get through a variety of stress-inducing situations.

Believe it or not, acting as if you have self-confidence can extend your "comfort zone." That's important to people lacking in self-confidence or self-esteem. According to Leary,

"Over time, the more uncomfortable or scary situations you force your way through by faking it a little, the less you will need to fake it. Each time, your self-esteem and self-confidence are naturally raised a notch or two." [2] Of course, there are instances of going to an extreme, forcing one's self through a very difficult situation despite the anxiety: the famous dance scene from the movie *Napoleon Dynamite* comes to mind. In order to help his friend, Pedro, who is running for class president of their high school, Napoleon alone takes center stage at the school-wide assembly and does an unrehearsed, unchoreographed dance in front of an auditorium full of his disaffected classmates. This audience at first starts out quite unreceptive, sitting stone-silent and staring at him.

We can all relate to this feeling Napoleon must have endured. We all sometimes have feelings of nervousness and intense pressure when facing certain situations. Jon Heder, the actor who plays Napoleon, describes the climactic moment of the film: "Everything leads up to this. . . . This has to be the moment where he lands a victory." Napoleon bets it all—and wins. He ends up getting cheers and then even a standing ovation (and Pedro gets elected!).[3]

Jon Gary Miller, who holds a degree in Dance–InterArts Technology, wrote in his article "The Napoleon Dynamite Dance Scene," that "the moral of the story is that having the courage to express your full self is both the scariest thing and the most wonderful thing in the world." The message is that we too can conquer our fears and build our self-esteem—if we face them.[4]

Thankfully, we don't necessarily have to go the route of the all-or-nothing gamble like Napoleon when it comes to dancing. We have the more comfortable option to take things slowly. We can take lessons with others who likely share some of the same hesitations and concerns as we have, and who are at a similar skill level as well. We interviewed Dyanne, a professional West Coast Swing instructor and competitor. She talked about her feelings when she was learning to dance. "When I was younger and first came to dancing, I was very very shy. I'm still quiet, but the dancing and the teaching of dance has connected me with people who support me. It's helped me with my confidence.

Now I can take that and apply it in other parts of my life. When I talk to one of my co-workers or my boss, I've become very good at explaining. As a dance teacher, I have had to learn to explain things in different ways, because the same explanation doesn't always work for different people. Now I'm more confident and my communication has gotten a lot easier and a lot clearer." As her abilities grew, so did her confidence.

When social dancers achieve a certain level of success, their self-esteem along with their confidence often improves.

So, there is a flip-side to the catch–22. That is, dance builds your confidence, and confidence builds your dance. The smart way to approach it: floortime is your friend. Simply stated, the more time you spend dancing, the better you get and the better you feel, both on and off the floor.

19   NO PAINING, YES GAINING (ON MENTAL HEALTH AND DEPRESSION!)

THE STORY

Joe is 62, extremely fit, and an avid dancer. His favorites are West Coast Swing and Country 2-Step. He is trim and muscular; he looks like he's ready to run a marathon. He is recently married, just celebrated his first year, and he is very happy. He's been dancing for about two-and-a-half years.

He first started dancing to improve his social life. He found he liked it and it got him out of his shell. When he first started, it was tough. Everything hurt and he wondered if he was too old to dance. But, he liked the music and he decided to take a private lesson. He contemplated quitting at various points, but he had found a dance partner and the two kept each other going.

He has mastered dancing enough now that it has become his regular aerobic workout. It allows him exercise, creativity and fun. Most importantly, it is good for his mental as well as physical health.

Joe describes himself as a recovering alcoholic; he has not had a drink in 25 years. Prone to depression, dance has been a huge help.

Not only does the movement contribute to his elevated mood, the fun he has doing it is also a huge help. He used to be very self-conscious dancing, but now he is much better both with his dancing and his confidence. He knows dance is providing the gift of health and wellbeing. He often dances at a place where he has seen people in their 80s, 90s, and even 100s dancing and that provides him with continued motivation and inspiration.

DANCING CURES DEPRESSION? REALLY?

It's no secret exercise is good for you, but it does actually relieve depression. Studies have been proving this over and over again for decades to the point it's almost common knowledge.

Better than Zoloft? Yep!

In *Understanding Depression*, a recent Harvard Medical School Special Health Report, doctors explain the benefits of exercise on depression, and site a study that shows regular exercise is at least as effective as antidepressants, such as Zoloft. For patients with depression who need or wish to avoid drugs, exercise might be an acceptable substitute for antidepressants. Even better, a follow-up to that study found the positive effects of exercise lasted longer than those of antidepressants.[1]

In a similar study, researchers found 30 minutes of brisk exercise three times a week is just as effective as drug therapy in relieving the symptoms of major depression in the short term, and continued exercise greatly reduces the chances of the depression returning.[2]

Another recent study explained directly this phenomenon of happiness cultivated by dancing. Researchers discovered the Argentine Tango worked as well as mindfulness meditation for relieving stress and depression, if not better. In the study, 66 participants were divided into three groups. One group took Tango classes, the other was assigned to meditate and the third was placed on a waiting list. Depression levels were reduced for both the Tango and meditation groups. Interestingly, only the Tango group achieved significantly reduced stress levels.[3]

HOW EXACTLY DOES EXERCISE WORK TO OVERCOME DEPRESSION?

The answer is endorphins. These are chemicals that have been naturally occurring within us for millennia, but have only started to be understood since the 1970s. Scientists discovered the human body makes it's own version of morphine, and named these chemicals accordingly: "endorphins" was coined by combining the words *endogenous*, meaning "proceeding from within; derived internally," and the pain-killer *morphine*. The researchers combined the *endo* from endogenous and the *orphin* from morphine together to describe these newly discovered chemicals, endorphins, the body's self-made feel-good drugs.[4]

Endorphins pretty much work as advertised by their names. They are analgesics our bodies produce naturally. They kick in when we exercise intensely for an "endorphin rush" or a "runner's high." However, they are elevated and then stick around for higher and sustained feelings of happiness and wellbeing with regular, moderate exercise. Again, studies show that's just about 30 minutes a day a few times a week.

SO HOW COME EVERYBODY ISN'T EXERCISING REGULARLY AND FEELING GREAT?

As you know, it's tough to stick to exercising. It is statistically likely that you have started and then abandoned a workout plan. According to the IHRSA (International Health, Racquet & Sportsclub Association), 67 percent of the people who have gym memberships *never* use them.[5] Hundreds of thousands of people enthusiastically begin well-thought-out programs of diets and exercise, only to drop them a few weeks or a couple of months later. Why is that?

Why *do* people keep failing with their diets and exercise? It's pretty simple, really. It's too hard to keep going, and it's really *not much fun*. Ever look around the gym at the faces in the weight room or the aerobics studio? How about the face of a runner? It's tough to find anyone smiling or looking the least bit pleased in these situations. That's because they're not particularly happy in the moment. Most people who are working out are in it for the secondary effect. In other words, they are taking their medicine because they know it's good for them, but they're not enjoying the taste of that medicine; they do it only for the cumulative benefit of good health and wellbeing they know it provides.

Unfortunately for many, this delayed-gratification-benefit of good health is simply not enough to overcome the unpleasantness, hassle and pain of regular exercise. Hence, the very high dropout rate.

DANCING IS THE ANSWER!

We won't repeat ourselves (too much) regarding the multiple benefits of dancing. This book is filled with them already. We'll just say this: Because dancing is fun, social, and relatively inexpensive and has a very low rate of injury, it's much easier for many people to stick with it.

BUT IS DANCING REALLY EVEN A DECENT WORKOUT?

In a word, yes.

The World DanceSport Federation (WDSF) refers to lead and follow dancing as sport, and its dancers as athletes. The International Olympic Committee agrees, having granted Ballroom dancing full recognition as a sport in 1997.[6]

According to the WDSF, "Choosing dance as a low-impact exercise regime to improve fitness is guaranteed to produce good results for people of all ages. In dance, hands, arms, legs, and head are continuously exerting forces in different directions—all at the same time. Dance can be one of the most complete cardiovascular and aerobic workouts. It is mentally engaging and physically demanding. And it is never dull, repetitive movement."[7]

Dr. Jill McNitt-Gray, professor of kinesiology and biological sciences at the University of Southern California, was asked by ABC's *Dancing with the Stars* to come on the show and explain some of the findings of recent scientific research regarding the level of fitness of dancers. She confirms: "Dancers are some of the toughest athletes in the world."[8]

The good news is you don't have to be a professional dancer to get the benefits from dancing. Among the many gains one can enjoy from dancing, the mental health component may be the greatest.

20 SOARING WITH THE EAGLES

IN 1898, SIX theatre owners came together to discuss a musicians' strike. Once they negotiated a way to handle the strike, they realized how productive coming together to hash things out could be, and they decided to form an organization called "The Order of Good Things." They held their meetings at a local theatre, and it became a social time with beer and music. As it grew, they took the American bald eagle as their official emblem and changed their name to "The Fraternal Order of Eagles." [1]

Most of the early members were actors, stagehands and playwrights who traveled across the United States and Canada and were responsible for the rapid growth of the organization. The organization is credited with the impetus for Social Security, ending age discrimination in the labor force, providing money for medical research and helping children with disabilities. Distinguished members included Billy Ray Cyrus, Jimmy Durante, Bob Hope, John F. Kennedy, Arnold Palmer, Eleanor Roosevelt, Franklin Delano Roosevelt, Theodore Roosevelt, and Harry S. Truman, just to name a few.[2]

An "aerie" is the name for the nest of a bird of prey. That is the name of the Eagles' official lodges. There are 1600 Aeries scattered across the United States and Canada.[3]

When you walk into the Eagles Lodge in Medford, Oregon, you feel you are entering a different world, reminiscent of the 1950s (in a good way). It is very welcoming, the drinks are inexpensive, and the patrons, mostly who are made up of retirees, are dressed to the nines and enjoying themselves immensely. When the music plays, everyone is up and dancing. They graciously agreed to let us interview a few of their members. This involved taking them momentarily away from their enjoyment of dancing to the live band which continued to belt out favorites while we chatted in the lounge.

THE STORIES:

MAGGIE

Maggie is a 91-year-old woman who has been ballroom dancing her whole life. As a child, she learned how to dance from her brothers. Her husband was not an avid dancer, so throughout her married life they only danced about once a month. He passed away many years ago, and after that her dancing picked up.

She notes her balance is excellent and so is her mind, which she attributes to dancing. She is in excellent health. She dances two to three times a week when she can get a ride to the dance hall. She considers frequent dancing as regular exercise for her physical health and card playing for her brain health. [Although we note the dancing is actually much better for her cognitive function, we refrained from chiding Maggie on this point.] At the Eagles, she has found community and an active social life as a result of ballroom dancing.

GEORGE

Now a spry 91-year-old, George played in a dance band when he was only 17. He saw the pretty girls on the dance-floor and decided it would be more fun to be with them rather than stuck on the stage. Not surprisingly, that inspired him to teach himself to dance.. Jitterbugging was his favorite, a dance he learned while he was in the service.

He became a public school teacher and then a school principal. He met his wife at a dance club where she worked as a cashier. She was 11 years older than he was. They danced together often, and had a great life. She died at the age of 96. At the Eagles Lodge, he found Jeanne, and they now dance five days a week.

George was slowed down a bit by prostate cancer and two heart attacks, but received good treatment and a good bill of health, and so is now back on his feet. He attributes his recovery to dancing and a love of health food. He enjoys having the music dictate the dance he chooses to do. For George, dance is a way of life. He feels it allows him to help others to get the most out of their lives as well.

JEANNE

George's partner is a self-described "doer", a trim 79-year-old woman with a twinkle in her eye. "I live to dance!" she exclaims. As we sit and talk to her it's clear. Even while seated, she can't stop moving to the music. She has danced her whole life and has no plans to ever stop. Her family was musical and sang and danced, and her father was her main dance teacher. She finds dance the healthiest thing in the world, and she dances as often as she can. Dancing is how she gets her exercise, and because she does it so often—she dances for at least two hours, five days a week—she is in great shape. She and George both love dancing Swing together; it's their favorite dance, but they dance just about every number and seem to love them all. Jeanne and George are a couple now and have a wonderful romance going on. They've been dancing up a storm for the last six years, and they don't see themselves stopping any time soon.

RUDY

When we saw him dancing with such precision and joy, we knew we had to talk to him. Sitting across the table, we'd swear Rudy wasn't 70; we were shocked to find out he was just about to turn 80. He danced and competed in dance as a child in his hometown of Dusseldorf, Germany. His wife, Suzanne, is 71-years-old, from Norway. (She was vacationing in Europe when we spoke with Rudy, due back in just a couple more weeks.) During his childhood and throughout his adult life, Rudy was somehow involved with dance, either actually doing it himself or bringing it to others, producing cabaret shows around the United States for audiences from Los Angeles to New York. Now "retired," he works part-time as a real estate broker.

Rudy and Suzanne (when she is back from Europe) dance almost every night. She loves to dance, and he feels that has helped their relationship, keeping them literally connected over the years. It is also their main form of exercise. Both are quite fit, both physically and mentally, and Rudy credits their regular dancing for this success.

For them, as for George and Jeanne, dancing is a way of life; they do not have to force themselves to do it, but rather it is something they look forward to. His advice: "If you are so inclined (or even if you are not!) just get up and dance. If you can count to three, you can do it, so you have no excuses!"

Experts and Evidence

You don't need an official study to know the harsh reality is that aging is the ultimate undoing of life and it will eventually kill you. In some ways, it's a deadly disease with which we're all afflicted, and there is no cure. As Jim Morrison voiced and then emphatically proved, "No one here gets out alive." Of course, dying at 27, one could argue in some ways, he got out easy. But, let's assume we'll take the long way home, and that we want to live as long and as well as we can.

A study (cited earlier in this work) was done looking at a group of elderly amateur dancers, each of whom been doing ballroom dance regularly for at least 16 years. They were compared to a non-dancing control group. The dancers were far superior when it came to multiple factors including cognitive performance, reaction times, posture, balance, and motor performance. Dancing had helped them to maintain important functions of the mind and body.

What we're looking for is successful aging, and that is what this study concluded. Dance has extensive benefits that make it a perfect activity to promote.[4]

Successful aging is what our friends from the Eagles have been proving for years. They are living right and living well, and a huge part of their success is due to dance. Although Medford, Oregon, is a relatively small city, it is, in many ways, not unique to other American cities: a significant portion of its population is elderly, and within that elderly population, people who dance are demonstrating better-than-average health and a higher quality of life than people who don't dance.

We'll close this chapter with not another quote, but a title from another research-based journal article. You can get the entire gist of it without bothering to read any further: "Dancing Combines the Essence for Successful Aging."[5] There. We just saved you some time. Now go use it wisely; *dance!*

"Nothing truly worthwhile is easy—
but your happiness and health are truly worthwhile."

—ROBIN MILLER AND DAVE KAHN

Afterward

WE HOPE YOU use this book to live a healthy and happy and long life. In each part we've offered some insight and motivation to achieve these goals.

In Part I, *The Basics*, we gave you a background of the most commonly challenging systems. With this knowledge, you now have a better understanding of how your heart, your gut and your brain work. In addition, you have information to improve communication and create a relationship—more of a collaboration—with your doctor.

In Part II, *What's New?* we offered some specifics about how you can live longer, avoid or cure depression, and some options beyond traditional medication to lift your mood. Our view is, if you can feel better with a change in diet or with specific foods and vitamins rather than with drugs, do it. However, we don't think drugs are evil. Some definitely can improve your quality of life, including the quality of your sex life.

In Part III, we focused on losing weight in a healthy, sustainable way: the *UnDiet*, also known as the *Teid Diet*. Distilled down to its most elemental message, once you learn how to consistently eat better and move more, you'll be able to maintain a healthy weight and attain fitness.

In Part IV, we taught you how to dance. Well, we taught you many reasons why you *should* be dancing. We truly believe dancing is one of the best things you can possibly do for your body, mind and spirit. We know if more people were aware of all the benefits, they would be dancing and the world would be a healthier, happier place.

We are confident if you make the effort and follow the precepts based on the information we've offered in this book—even if you only choose to embrace parts of it—you will enjoy the ultimate wealth: health and you will live a happier and longer life. You will truly be *well-healed*.

Will You Please Do Us A Favor?

If you enjoyed *Healed*, would you please mind taking a moment to write a review on Amazon? Even a short comment will help. It would mean so much to us!

If you or someone you love is trying to find the right doctor, the best solutions to staying healthy and fit or trying to find activities that address total body wellness, please send them a copy of this book.

If you would like to order copies for your company, groups of friends or business please go to wellhealed.net and order.

If you would like to access new materials and updates, follow us on Facebook at SOswing: WCSwing in S. Oregon or Dr. Robin Miller's professional page.

You will find websites for dance events around that country where you can learn and dance to your heart's content (and health)!

It is time to enjoy a healthy life and dance!

Cheat Sheet For Your Doctor Visit

FIRST:

➥ Check out this website to find an Integrative Medicine practitioner: www.integrativemedicine.arizona.edu/alumni.html.

THEN:

➥ Go to the AskMD an app for your phone or computer. It will help you organize your thoughts and give your doctor a print out of your concerns and possible diagnoses.

➥ For brain and overall health, you may want to ask for the MTHFR test. It can be done with a simple blood test. It is covered by Medicare and many insurance companies.

➥ For gut health, discuss probiotics.

SPECIFICS TO ASK FOR:

❏ Other blood tests that you may want to have done include: Fasting blood sugar, Vitamin D, B12, magnesium and zinc that are important basic labs for assessment of general health and the NMR lipoprofile and possibly TMAO.

❏ If you are suffering from PTSD, EMDR may be of benefit

❏ If you are in the need of antidepressants, consider asking your doctor to do a GeneSight test.

❏ Find a good compounding pharmacy if you are interested in Viagra for women.

FOR OVERALL HEALTH:

❏ Come up with a reasonable eating and exercise plan that works for you with the help of your doctor.

❏ Have a physical exam before you start a dance program.

❏ If you are out of shape, start your dance program slowly. Then . . .

❏ **Find a place to dance, get some good shoes and go!**

Dance CONVENTIONS LOCATED AROUND THE US

We love West Coast Swing, and many of these amazing events offer WCS—along with a lot of other very fun dances.

Listed are weekend-long events with LOTS of dancing, instruction, competitions and shows. For more information, schedules and specific dates, we recommend you visit the event site, but also look at the World Swing Dance Council web site: worldsdc.com. There you will find all the links to the events below as well as to many other dance events from the US and all over the world!

LATE DECEMBER INTO JANUARY:

THE PALM SPRINGS NEW YEARS SWING DANCE CLASSIC
peoplewhodance.com

IN JANUARY:

MONTEREY SWING FEST: CA
centralcoastswingdance.com

SWINGCOUVER: VANCOUVER, CANADA
swingcouver.com
(Yes, we know this one's not technically in the US, but it's really close.)

DERBY CITY SWING, LOUISVILLE, KY
derbycityswing.com

IN FEBRUARY:

CHARLOTTE WESTIE FEST: NC
charlottewestivefest.com

DANCE CAMP CHICAGO: IL
swingincountry.net

CAPITAL SWING DANCE: SACRAMENTO, CA
capitalswingconvention.com

SWEETHEART SWING CLASSIC: TAMPA BAY, FL
sweetheartswingclassic.com

ROSE CITY SWING: PORTLAND, OR
rosecityswingevents.com

5280: AURORA-DENVER, CO
5280westival.com

IN MARCH:

HIGH DESERT DANCE CLASSIC: LANCASTER, CA
highdesertdancelassic.com

MAD JAM: BALTIMORE, MD
atlanticdancejam.com

THE BOSTON TEA PARTY: BOSTON, MA
teapartyswings.com

NOVICE INVITATIONAL HUSTON: TX
novice-invitational.com

SWING OVER ORLANDO: FL
swingoverorlando.com

CITY OF ANGELS: CA
cityofangelesswing.com

SEATTLE EASTER SWING: SEATTLE, WA
easterswing.org

IN APRIL:

SAN DIEGO DANCE FESTIVAL, CA
sandiegodancefestival.com

SWING DANCE AMERICA: LAKE GENEVA, WISCONSIN
swingdanceamerica.com

SEATTLE EASTER SWING: SEATTLE, WA
easterswing.org
(Like Easter, this one moves around.)

IN MAY:

SWING DIEGO: SAN DIEGO, CA
swingdiego.com

SWINGIN' INTO SPRING: HARTFORD, CT
sis.dkkenm.com

THE TEXAS CLASSIC: HOUSTON, TX
thetexasclassic.com

SOSWING CONVENTION: MEDFORD, OR
soswing.org

USA GRAND NATIONAL DANCE CHAMPIONSHIP, ATLANTA, GA
usagrandnationals.com

FREZNO DANCE CLASSIC: FREZNO, CA
freznodanceclassic.weebly.com

THE SHOW-ME SHOWDOWN: SPRINGFIELD, MO
theshowmeshowdown.com

IN JUNE:

MICHIGAN CLASSIC: DEARBORN, MI
miciganclassicswing.com

ORANGE BLOSSOM DANCE FESTIVAL: ORLANDO, FL
orangeblossomdance.net

JACK AND JILL O'RAMA: ORANGE COUNTY, CA
jackandjillorama.com

DANCE N PLAY: REDMOND, OR
dancenplay.com

COLORADO COUNTRY CLASSIC: DENVER, CO
coloradocountryclassic.net

LIBERTY SWING DANCE CHAMPIONSHIPS: NEW BRUNSWICK, NJ
libertyswing.com

WILD WILD WESTIE: DALLAS, TX
wildwildwestie.com

INDY DANCE EXPLOSION: INDIANAPOLIS, IN
indydancex.com

IN JULY:

BIG APPLE COUNTRY DANCE & NY SWING CONGRESS: NEWARK, NJ
bigapplecountrydance.com

PHOENIX 4TH OF JULY SWING CONVENTION: PHOENIX, AZ
phoenixjuly4swingconvention.com

PORTLAND DANCE FESTIVAL: PORTLAND, OR
portlanddancefestival.com

FLORIDA DANCE MAGIC: JUPITER, FL
floridadancemagic.com

DANCE MARTI GRAS: NEW ORLEANS, LA
dancemartigras.com

SACRAMENTO ALL SWING: CA
sacramentoallswing.com

PALM SPRINGS SUMMER DANCE CAMP CLASSIC, CA
jaybayam.com

SWINGTIME IN THE ROCKIES: DENVER, CO
swingtimeintherockies.com

IN AUGUST:

ARIZONA DANCE CLASSIC: PHOENIX
arizonadanceclassic.com

MIDWEST WESTIE FEST: KANSAS CITY, KS
miswestwestiefest.com

LONESTAR INVITATIONAL: AUSTIN, TX
lonstarcountrydance.com

SWINGTACULAR: THE GALACTIC OPEN: SANTA CLARA, CA
dancegeekproductions.com

SWING FLING: HERDON, VA
swingfling.com

CHICAGOLAND DANCE FESTIVAL, IL
chicagolanddancefestival.com

SUMMER HUMMER: FRAMINGHAM, MA
dancepros.net

SOUTH BAY DANCE FLING: SAN JOSE, CA
southbaydancefling.com

IN SEPTEMBER:

TRILOGY SWING: DURHAM, NC
swingtrilogy.com

UPSTATE DANCE CHALLENGE: ALBANY, NY
upstatedancechallenge.com

PHILLY SWING CLASSIC: PA
phillyswings.com

MEET ME IN ST. LOUIS SWING DANCE CHAMPIONSHIPS: MO
meetmeinstlouissdc.com

BRIDGETOWN SWING: PORTLAND, OR
portlandswing.org/bts/

IN OCTOBER:

BOOGIE BY THE BAY: SAN FRANCISCO, CA
boogiebythebay.org

IN NOVEMBER:

MOUNTAIN MAGIC: LAKE TAHOE, CA
michelledance.com

SEA TO SKY: SEATTLE, WA
seatoskydance.com

THE US OPEN: BURBANK, CA
usopenswing.com

IN DECEMBER:

THE AFTER PARTY: IRVINE, CA
tapwcs.com

End NOTES

CHAPTER 1

1. CDC 2009

CHAPTER 2

1. CDC 2008

2. Biswas et al. 2015

CHAPTER 3

1. Heidelbaugh et al. 2015

2. Berg et al. 2015

3. Rubio-Tabia 2012

4. CDF 2016

5. Natural Food Revolution 2015

6. Dupont 2013

7. Triantafillidis 2009

8. Drossman 2011

9. Saito-Loftus 2011

10. Tan, Hammond and Joseph ,2005

CHAPTER 4

1. Bryan 2014

2. NIA-NIH 2015

3. NIA-NIH 2015

4. Feart et al. 2009

5. Lim et al. 2005

6. Beeri 2008

7. McClean et al. 2011

8. Relkin 2014

9. Bredesen 2014

10. Iwasaki et al. 1990

11. NINDS 2016

12. Sian 1999

13. Shin 2012

14. Toovey, Jick and Meier 2011

15. Takahashi 1999

16. Weaver et al. 2012

17. NIH/CDC 2016

18 NINDS 2016

CHAPTER 5

1. Aubert 2008

2. Gladstone 2012

3. Ameur et al. 2011

4. Sinha 2014

5. Horvath 2015

6. Wilcox 2010

7. Fata 2014

8. Shurkin 1992

9. Paffenbarger 1978

10. Vaillant 2012

CHAPTER 6

1. Zivin et al. 2007

2. CDC 2014

3. Bornfeld 2011

4. Barbui et al. 2011

5. Morton 2000

6. Young 2008

7. Guaraldi 1993

8. Papakostas 2012

9. Papakostas 2012

10. Shapiro 2014

11. EMDR Institute 2015

12. Galizia 2014

13. Blumenthal et al. 2007

14. Baily 2000

15. Willey 2014

16. Seppala et al. 2013

17. Ahmed 2013

18. NIH 2016

19. Kjaergaard et al. 2012

20. Gupta 2014

21. Wang et al. 2013

22. Appleton et al. 2006

23. Montgomery and Richardson 2009

24. Antypa 2008

CHAPTER 7

1. Sofi 2008

2. Lucas et al. 2013

3. Zagursky 2014

4. Hilimire et al. 2015

5. Bercik 2011

6. Turnbaugh 2006

7. Clarke, Murphy, O'Sullivan et al. 2014

8. Cerdá, Pérez-Santiago et al. 2016

9. Cronin, Molloy, Shanahan. 2016

10. Kang, Jeraldo, Kurti et al. 2014

11. Hicks. 2010.

12. Suez, Korem, Zeevi et al. 2014.

CHAPTER 8

1. Dong 2011

2. Ross et al. 2000

3. Eskelinen et al. 2009

4. Lucas et al. 2013.

5. Terry, Doumas and Wing 2009

6. Kim et al. 2012

7. Hedstrom et al. 2015

8. Glicksman et al. 2014

9. Ding et al. 2014

10. Smith et al. 2006

11. Kennedy et al. 2016

12. AICR 2015

13. Merritt et al. 2015

14. Tang et al. 2010

15. Loftfield et al. 2013

16. Schmit et al. 2016

17. Ding et al. 2015

18. Bonaa et al. 1988.

19. Sorond et al. 2013

20. Sahib et al. 2010

21. Sunni and Latif 2014

22. Kwok et al. 2014

23. Buijsse et al. 2006

24. Djousse et al. 2011

25. Djousse et al. 2010

26. Galleano et al. 2009.

27. Williams, Tamburic and Lally. 2009

28. Ames 2000

29. Koytchev et al. 1999

30. Wolbling 1994

31. Guggenheim, Wright and Zwickey 2014

32. Jong and Birmingham 1992

33. Chen 2010

34. Borchers 1999

35. Dai 2015

36. Torkelson 2012

37. Anderson 2010

38. Vandeven, Nghiem 2012

39. Wong, et al. 2012

40. Sabaratnam et al. 2013

41. Nagano et al. 2010

CHAPTER 9

1. Society for Personality and Social Psychology. 2015

2. Stulberg et al. 2008

3. Berman et al. 2003

4. Lindau, et al. 2007

5. Santoro, Komi 2009

6. Takahashi, Okada, Ozaki 2000

7. Tahereh, Najafi 2013

8. Dmitrovic et al. 2013

CHAPTER 10

1. Jampolis 2011

2. WHO 2016

3. Mann et al. 2007

4. Fidles et al. 2015

5. Singh et al. 2015

6. Leech 2015

7. Yang 2010

8. Gardener 2012

9. Falbe 2013

10. Rains et al. 2015

11. Lennert et al. 2011

12. Lytx 2014

13. Jakubowicz et al. 2013

14. Smithsonian 2007

15. Shimizu et al. 2014

16. Hermans et al. 2012

17. Wing and Jeffrey 1999

18. Christakis and Fowler 2007

19. Spellman 2016

20. Dulloo et al.1997

21. Ludwig and Friedman. 2014

22. Spellman 2016

PART IV

1. J Giles 2005, Vaillant 2012

CHAPTER 11

1. Snowdon 1996

2. Verghese et al. 2003

3. Brown, Martinez and Parsons 2006

4. Raji 2010

5. Verghese et al. 2003

6. Hackney and Earhart 2009

7. Hackney 2014

8. Hackney 2009

9. Hurt et al. 1998

10. Teixeira, et. al. 2012.

CHAPTER 12

1. Bray 2012

2. CDC 2016

3. Nagashima et al. 2010

4. Mangeri et al. 2014

5. DanceUK 2016

6. Howley 2015

7. Colberg et al. 2010

CHAPTER 13

1. CDC 2015
2. Huppertz 2015
3. Allender, Cowburn and Foster 2006
4. Guidarini et al. 2013
5. Belardinelli et al. 2008

CHAPTER 14

1. NIH 2013
2. CDC 2016
3. CDC 2016, NIH 2015, Sollitto 2016
4. Tartar 2016, Doll 2015
5. Kattenstroth et al. 2010
6. Gomes et al. 2014
7. Kattenstroth et al. 2013

CHAPTER 15

1. IOF 2016,
2. Johnell and Kanis 2006
3. NOF 2016
4. CDC 2015

CHAPTER 16

1. Brown, et al. 2012
2. Goodill et al. 2011

CHAPTER 17

1. Henry 2013
2. Knaus 2008
3. ADMT 2016
4. Bräuniger 2016
5. Dance Pizazz 2015

CHAPTER 18

1. Leary 2001
2. Leary 2001.
3. Herder 2012
4. Miller 2010

CHAPTER 19

1. Blumenthal, Smith and Hoffman 2012
2. Blumenthal et al. 1999
3. Pinniger et al. 2012
4. Miller-Keane 2007
5. IHRSA 2015
6. M.P. 2015
7. WDSF 2016
8. McNitt-Gray 2008

CHAPTER 20

1. FOE 2016
2. FOE 2016
3. FOE 2016
4. Kattenstroth 2010
5. Olsson 2012

Sources

(AICR) American Institute for Cancer Research.www.aicr.org/press/press-releases/2015/liver-cancer-report-new-links-emerge-coffee-protective-obesity-risk.html

(ADTA) American Dance Therapy Association. 2016 FAQs: What Is Dance Movement Therapy? www.adta.org/faqs/

Ahmad I, T. Mirza, K. Qadee, et al. "Vitamin B6: deficiency diseases and methods of analysis." Pak J Pharm Sci. 26(5):1057-69.

Allender, S. G. Cowburn, C. Foster. 2006. "Understanding participation in sport and physical activity among children and adults: a review of qualitative studies." Oxford Journals.(21)6:826-835.

Ames M. 2000. Herpes: Comprehensive treatment strategy. Int J Integra Med. 2(5):6-9

Ameur, A., J. Stewart, C. Freyer, et al. 2011. "Ultra-Deep Sequencing of Mouse Mitochondrial DNA: Mutational Patterns and Their Origins." PLoS Genet 7(3):20-28.

Angosta, A., R Serafica, S. Moonie. 2015. "Measuring Enjoyment of Ballroom Dancing in Filipino Americans Using the Physical Activity Enjoyment Scale." Asian Pacific Island Nursing Journal (2)2.

Appleton KM, R.C.Hayward, D. Gunnell, et al. 2006. "Effects of n-3 long-chain polyunsaturated fatty acids on depressed mood: systematic review of published trials." Am J Clin Nutr.84:1308-1316.

Antypa, N. A.J. Van der Does, A.H. Smelt et al. 2008. "Omega-3 fatty acids (fish-oil) and depression-related cognition in healthy volunteers." J Psychopharmacol.(7):831-40

Aubert, G., P.M. Lansdorp. 2008. "Telomeres and aging." Physiol Rev. 88(2):557-79.

Barbui, C., A. Cipriani, V. Patel, et al. 2011. "Efficacy of antidepressants and benzodiazepines in minor depression: systematic review and meta-analysis." Br J Psychiatry. 198(1):11-6,sup 1.

Bercik P, E. Denou, J. Collins, et al. 2011 "The intestinal microbiota affect central levels of brain-derived neurotropic factor and behavior in mice." Gastroenterology.141(2):599-609.

Beeri MS, J Schmeidler, J. Silverman et al. 2008. "Insulin in combination with other diabetes medication is associated with less Alzheimer neuropathology." Neurology 71:750–757.

Belardinelli, R., F. Lacalaprice, C. Ventrella, et al. 2008. "Waltz Dancing in Patients With Chronic Heart Failure." Circulation: Heart Failure. 1:107-114.

Berman, J. L. Berman, S.M. Toler, et al. 2003. "Safety and Efficacy of Sildenafil Citrate for the Treatment of Female Sexual Arousal Disorder: A Double-Blind, Placebo Controlled Study." The Journal of Urology. 170: pp 2333-2338.

Beth Israel Deaconess Medical Center and Harvard Medical School Teaching Hospital, 2016. "Week 1: The Science of Set Point." www.bidmc.org/YourHealth/BIDMCInteractive/ Break-Through-Your-Set-Point/Week-One-The-Science-of-Set-Point.aspx

Blumenthal JA, MA Babyak, P.M. Doraiswamy, et al. 2007. "Exercise and pharmacotherapy in the treatment of major depressive disorder." Psychosom Med. 69(7):587–96.

Blumenthal, J.A., P.J. Smith, B.M. Hoffman. 2012. "Is Exercise a Viable Treatment for Depression?" ACSMs Health Fit J. 16(4):14-21.

Bonaa, K., E. Arnesen, D.S. Thelle and O.H. Forde. 1988. Coffee and cholesterol: is it all in the brewing? The Tromsø Study. BMJ. 297(6656): 1103–1104.

Borchers A.T., J.S. Stern, R.M. Hackman, et al. 1999. "Mushrooms, tumors, and immunity." Proc Soc Exp Biol Med. 221:281-293.

Borges, E.G., R.G. Vale, S.A. Cader, et al. 2010. "Postural balance and falls in elderly nursing home residents enrolled in a ballroom dancing program." Front Aging Neuroscience 2:31.

Bornfield, S. 2011. Antidepressants most popular prescription medication in U.S. Las Vegas Review Journal: www.reviewjournal.com/life/health/antidepressants-most-popular-prescription-medication-us

Bräuniger, Iris, Ph.D. 2016. "It Can Help Substance Abuse, PTSD, Shyness, and More." www.anxiety.org/what-is-dance-movement-therapy.

Bray G.A. 2012 "Exercise for Weight Loss." JAMA. 307(24):2641-2642

Bredesen, D.E. 2014. "Reversal of cognitive decline: A novel therapeutic program." Aging. 6(9): 707-717.

Brown, J.C., K. Winters-Stone, L, A. Lee, K.H. Schmitz. 2012. Cancer, Physical Activity and Exercise. BCompr Physio. 2(4): 2775-2809.Brown S.B., M.J. Martinez, L.M. Parsons. 2006. "The neural basis of human dance." Cerebral Cortex.16:1157–1167.

Buijsse, B. E.J. Feskens, D. Kromhout, et al. 2006. "Cocoa intake, blood pressure, and cardiovascular mortality: the Zutphen Elderly Study." Arch Intern Med. 27;166(4):411-7.

Byungsung, K.Y. Nam, J. Kim, et al. 2012. "Coffee Consumption and Stroke Risk: A Meta-analysis of Epidemiologic Studies." Korean Journal Family Medicine. 33(6): 356–365.

Cardoso, C.G., R.S. Gomides, A. C. C. Queiroz, et al. 2010. "Acute and chronic effects of aerobic and resistance exercise on ambulatory blood pressure." Clinics 65(3).

CDC (Centers for Disease Control and Prevention). 2008. "Disparities in Adult Awareness of Heart Attack Warning Signs and Symptoms—14 States, 2005." MMWR February 22, 2008 57(07): 175-179.

CDC. (Centers for Disease Control and Prevention.) 2009. "The Power of Prevention. Chronic Disease....the public health challenge of the 21st Century." www.cdc.gov/chronicdisease/pdf/2009-power-of-prevention.pdf

CDC (Centers for Disease Control and Prevention.) 2016. "Important facts about falls." www.cdc.gov/HomeandRecreationalSafety/Falls/adultfalls.html

CDC (Centers for Disease Control and Prevention.) 2015. "Nutrition, Physical Activity and Obesity, Data, Trends and Maps."

www.nccd.cdc.gov/NPAO_DTM/LocationSummary.aspx?statecode=94

www.cdc.gov/mentalhealth/basics/mental-illness/depression.htm

www.cdc.gov/traumaticbraininjury/pubs/tbi_report_to_congress.html 1999.

www.cdc.gov/nchs/fastats/exercise.htm 2015

CDF. 2016. "What is Celiac Disease?" www.celiac.org/celiac-disease/what-is-celiac-disease/

Cerdá, Pérez, B., M.,Pérez-Santiago, J, et. al. 2016. Gut Microbiota Modification: Another Piece in the Puzzle of the Benefits of Physical Exercise in Health? Front Physiology. 7:51

Chen J.T., K. Tominaga. Y. Sato et al. 2010. "Maitake mushroom (Grifola frondosa) extract induces ovulation in patients with polycystic ovary syndrome: a possible monotherapy and a combination therapy after failure with first-line clomiphene citrate." J Altern Complement Med. 16:1295-9.

Christakis, N.A., J.H. Fowler. 2007. The Spread of Obesity in a Large Social Network over 32 Years. N Engl J Med. 357:370-379.

Christensen, K., T.E. Johnson, J.W. Vaupel. 2006. "The quest for genetic determinants of human longevity: challenges and insights." Nat Rev Genet 7(6): 436–448.

Clarke, S.F., E.F. Murphy, O. O'Sullivan, et.al. 2014. Exercise and associated dietary extremes impact on gut microbial diversity. Gut. 63:1913-1920

Cohen SO, G.A.Walco. 1999. "Dance/Movement therapy for children and adolescents with cancer. Cancer Practice." 7(1):34-42.

Colberg, S.R., R. Sigal, B. Fernhall, et al. 2010. "Exercise and Type 2 Diabetes. Diabetes Care." 33(12) 147-167.

Coppen A., J. Bailey. 2000. Enhancement of the antidepressant action of fluoxetine by folic acid: a randomised, placebo controlled trial. J Affect Disord. 60(2):121-30.)

Constantino, D., C. Guaraldi. 2008 Effectiveness and safety of vaginal suppositories for the treatment of the vaginal atrophy in postmenopausal women: an open, non-controlled clinical trial. European Review for Medical and Pharmacological Sciences. 12: 411-416.

Cronin, O., MG Molloy, F. Shanahan. 2016 Exercise, fitness and the gut. Curr Opin Gastroenterol. 32:67-73.

Dance Pizazz, 2015. www.prweb.com/releases/2015/04/prweb12647601.htm

DanceUK. 2016. www.danceuk.org/resources/dance-facts/

Dash, S., G. Clarke, M. Berk, et al. 2015. "The Gut Microbiome and Diet in Psychiatry: Focus on Depression." Curr Opin Psychiatry. 28(1):1-6.

Ding, M.,A. Satija, S.N. Bhupathiraju, et al. 2015. "Association of Coffee Consumption with Total and Cause-Specific Mortality in Three Large Prospective Cohorts." Circulation. DOI: 10.1161/circulationaha.115.017341

Ding M., S.N Bhupathiraju, A. Satija, R.M.,van Dam, F.B. Hu .2014. Long-term coffee consumption and risk of cardiovascular disease: a systematic review and a dose-response meta-analysis of prospective cohort studies. Circulation. 129(6)643-59.

Djousse, L.,P.N. Hopkins, D.K. Arnett, et al. 2011. "Chocolate consumption is inversely associated with calcified atherosclerotic plaque in the coronary arteries: the NHLBI Family Heart Study." Clin Nutr. 2011 Feb;30(1):38-43

Dmitrovic, R., A.R. Kunselman, R.S. Legro, et al. 2013. "Sildenafil citrate in the treatment of pain in primary dysmenorrhea: a randomized controlled trial. Human Reproduction." Vol 0 (0):1-8.

Doll, J. 2015. "Powerlifting records at 85 years old." www.pinchercreekecho.com /2015/07/05/powerlifting-world-records-at-85-years-old

Dong, J., J. Zou, X.F. Yu. 2011. "Coffee drinking and pancreatic cancer risk: A meta-analysis of cohort studies." World J Gastroenterol. 17(9): 1204-1210.

Dulloo, A.G., J. Jacquet, L. Girardier, et al. 1997. "Poststarvation hyperphagia and body fat overshooting in humans: a role for feedback signals from lean and fat tissues." Am J Clin Nutr. 65(3):717-23.

Dupont, V. 2013. "GMO corn, soybeans dominate US market." www.phys.org/news/2013-06-gmo-corn-soybeans-dominate.html

Erickson, K.I., C.A. Raji, O.L. Lopez, et al. 2010. "Physical activity predicts gray matter volume in late adulthood: the Cardiovascular Health Study." Neurology. 75(16):1415-22.

Eskelinen, M.H., T. Ngandu, J. Tuomilehto, et al. 2009. "Midlife coffee and tea drinking and the risk of late-life dementia: a population-based CAIDE study." J Alzheimer's Disease. 16(1):85-91.

Fackelmann, K 2005. "Doing the tango keeps the brain in step, too." USA Today.

Falbe, J.,B. Rosner, W.C. Willett, et al. 2013. "Adiposity and Different Types of Screen Time." Pediatrics. 132(6): 1497–1505.

Feart C, et al. 2009. "Adherence to a Mediterranean diet, Cognitive Decline, and risk of Dementia." Journal of the American Medical Association 303: 638-648.

Fildes, A., J. Charlton, C. Rudisill, et al. 2015. "Probability of an Obese Person Attaining Normal Body Weight: Cohort Study Using Electronic Health Records." American Journal of Public Health. 105(9): 54-59.

FOE (Fraternal Order of the Eagles). 2016. www.foe.com/about.aspx

FRAC (Food Research & Action Center). 2015. "Obesity in the US." 2015. www.frac.org/initiatives/hunger-and-obesity/obesity-in-the-us/

Gardner, H. , T. Rundek, et al. 2012. "Diet Soft Drink Consumption Is Associated with an Increased Risk of Vascular Events in the Northern Manhattan Study." Journal of General Internal Medicine. 27 (9): 1120-1126.

Giles L.C., G.F. Glonek, M.A. Luszcz, G.R.Andrews. 2005. "Effect of social networks on 10-year survival in very old Australians: the Australian longitudinal study of aging." Journal of Epidemiology and Community Health. 59:574-9.

Glicksman J.T., S.G. Curhan, G.C. Curhan, et al. 2014. "A prospective study of caffeine intake and risk of incident tinnitus." American Journal of Medicine. Aug; 127(8):739-43.

Greer, T. 2013. "UAB ballroom dance study enrolling cancer survivors." UAB News.

Guggenheim, A.G., K.M. Wright, H.L. Zwickey. 2014. "Immune Modulation From Five Major Mushrooms: Application to Integrative Oncology." Integr Med (Encinitas). 13(1): 32–44.

Guidarini, F.C., I.C. Schenkel, V.V. Kessler, et al. 2013. "Ballroom dance: chronic responses on blood pressure in medicated hypertensives". RBCDH. 15:155.

Gupta, P. S. Tiwar, J. Haria, et al. 2014. "Relationship Between Depression and Vitamin C Status: A Study on Rural Patients From Western Uttar Pradesh in India." International Journal of Scientific Study. Vol 1 (4): 37-39.

Hackney, M. E., G.M. Earhart. 2009. "Effects of Dance on Movement Control in Parkinson's Disease: A Comparison of Argentine Tango and American Ballroom." Journal of Rehabilitation Medicine. 41(6): 475-481.

Harris, S. 2005. "Studies with Dancing, Computer Training, Show Ways to Maintain

Hogg, J., A. Diaz, M. Del Cid, et al. 2012. "An after-school dance and lifestyle education program reduces risk factors for heart disease and diabetes in elementary school children." J. Pediatric Endocrinology Metabolism. 25(0): 509-516.

Howley,E. 2015. www.calorielab.com/burned/?mo=se&gr=03&ti=dancing&q&wt=150&un=lb&kg=68

Horvath, S. 2015. "DNA methylation age of human tissues and cell types." Genome Biology. 16:96.

Huppertz C., M. Bartels, I.E. Jansen, et al. 2014. "A twin-sibling study on the relationship between exercise attitudes and exercise behavior." Behav Genet 2014 Jan;44(1):45-55

Hurt C. R.R. Rice,G.C. McIntosh, M.H. Thaut. 1998. "Rhythmic Auditory Stimulation in Gait Training for Patients with Traumatic Brain Injury." Journal of Music Therapy 35(4): 228-241.

(IHRSA) International Health, Racquet & Sportsclub Association, Annual Report, 2015. www.statisticbrain.com/gym-membership-statistics/

(IOF) International Osteoporosis Foundation. 2016. www.iofbonehealth.org/facts-statistics

Jakubowicz D., M. Barnea, J. Wainstein, O. Froy. 2013. "High Caloric intake at breakfast vs. dinner differentially influences weight loss of overweight and obese women." Obesity. 21(12):2504-12.

James, B.D., S.E. Leurgans, LE. Herbert, et al. 2014. "Contribution of Alzheimer disease to mortality in the United States." Neurology. 82(12): 1045-1050.

Jampolis, Dr. Melina. 2011. "Expert Q & A: Which Test Should I Trust When Measuring My Body Fat?" CNN. Diet and Fitness. www.cnn.com/2011/HEALTH/expert.q.a /09/30/body.fat.testing.jampolis/

Johnell O.,J.A. Kanis JA. 2006. "An estimate of the worldwide prevalence and disability associated with osteoporotic fractures." Osteoporos Int 17:1726.

Jong, S. C., J. M. Birmingham. 1992. "Medicinal benefits of the mushroom Ganoderma." Adv. Appl Microbiol. 37:101-134.

Kang, S.S., Jeraldo P. R., Kurti A., et al. (2014). Diet and exercise orthogonally alter the gut microbiome and reveal independent associations with anxiety and cognition. Mol. Neurodegener. 9:36.

Kattenstroth, J C., I. Kolankowska, T. Kalish, H.R, Dinse. 2010. "Superior Sensory, Motor, and Cognitive Performance in Elderly Individuals with Multi-Year Dancing Activities." Front Aging Neurosci. 2010; 2: 31.

Kattenstroth J.C., T. Kalisch, S. Holt, et al. 2013. "Six months of dance intervention enhances postural, sensorimotor, and cognitive performance in elderly without affecting cardio-respiratory functions." Front Aging Neurosci. 5:5.

Kattenstroth, J.C., T. Kalisch, I. Kolankowska, H. Dinse. 2011. "Balance, Sensorimotor, and Cognitive Performance in Long-Year Expert Senior Ballroom Dancers." Access to Research Journal of Aging Research: 2011: 10-20

Katzman R. 1993. "Education and the prevalence of dementia and Alzheimer's disease." Neurology. 43:13-20.

Kennedy, O.J., P. Roderick, R. Buchanan, et al. 2016. "Systematic review with meta-analysis: coffee consumption and the risk of cirrhosis." Aliment Pharmacol Ther. 43(5):562-74.

Keogh, J.W., A. Kilding, A. Pidgeon, et al. 2009. "Physical Benefits of Dancing for Healthy Older Adults: A Review." Journal of Aging and Physical Activity, 17: 1-23.

Kern, E., E. Chun, J. Schwartz. 2014. "The Breast Cancer Lifestyle Intervention Pilot Study." Journal of Cancer Therapy. 5:1031-1038.

Kim, S.E., M. Kim, Y.B. Ahn, et al. 2011. "Effect of Dance Exercise on Cognitive Function in Elderly Patients with Metabolic Syndrome: A Pilot Study." Journal of Sports Science Medicine. 10(4):671-678.

Kjaergaard, M., Waterloo, K., Wang, C.E, et al.2012. "Effect of vitamin D supplement on depression scores in people with low levels of serum 25-hydroxyvitamin D: nested case-control study and randomised clinical trial." Br J Psychiatry. 201(5): p. 360-8.

Knaus, W.J. 2008."The Cognitive Behavioral Workbook for Anxiety: A Step-by-Step Program." New Harbinger.

Knaus, B. 2012. "Overcoming Shyness and Social Anxieties, Science and Sensibility, Psychology Today." www.psychologytoday.com/blog/science-and-sensibility/201206/ overcoming-shyness-and-social-anxieties

Koch, S.C.,K. Morlinghaus, T. Fuchs. 2007. "The joy dance . Specific effects of a single dance intervention on psychiatric patients with depression." The Arts in Psychotherapy 34: 340–349.

Knopman, D.S. 2009 "Editorial: Mediterranean Diet no quick fix for mental decline." Journal of the American Medical Association. 303:686-687.

Koytchev R., R.G. Alken, S. Dundarov. 1999. "Balm mint extract (Lo-701) for topical treatment of recurring Herpes labialis." Phytomedicine. 1999; 6: 225-230

Kwok, C.S., S.. Boekholdt, M.H. Lenties, et al. 2014. "Habitual chocolate consumption and risk of cardiovascular disease among healthy men and women." Heart doi:10.1136/heartjnl-2014-307050

La Fata, G., P. Weber, M.H. Mohajeri.2014. "Effects of Vitamin E on Cognitive Performance during Ageing and in Alzheimer's Disease." Nutrients. 6(12):5453-5472.

Leary, M.
www1.cfnc.org/Home/Article.aspx?articleId=TKZjBonzsuebU8XAP2BPAX

Leech, J. 2015. "Thirteen Ways That Sugary Soda Is Bad for Your Health." Authority Nutrition. www.authoritynutrition.com/13-ways-sugary-soda-is-bad-for-you/

Lewis, S., C.H. Hennekens. 2015. Steven Lewis, Charles H. Hennekens. 2015. "Regular Physical Activity: Forgotten Benefits." The American Journal of Medicine, 128 (11): 1159-1262.

Lim, G.P.,F. Calon, T Morihara et al. 2005. "A diet enriched with omega-3 fatty acid docosahexaenoic acid reduces amyloid burden in an ages Alzheimer mouse model." J Neurosci. 25(12): 3032-40.

Lindau ST, Schumm LP. Laumann EO, Levinson W, O_Muircheartaigh CA, Waite LJ. A study of sexuality and health among older adults in the United States. N Engl J Med 2007;357:762-774.

Loftfield, E, N. Freedman, B.I. Graubard, et al. 2015. "Coffee Drinking and Cutaneous Melanoma Risk in the NIH-AARP Diet and Health Study." JNCI J Natl Cancer Inst. 107 (2): dju421 doi:10.1093/jnci/dju421

Lovatt, P. 2011. "Dance confidence, age and gender. Personality and Individual Differences." Vol. 50(5):668–672.

Lucas, M., E.J. O'Reilly, A. Pan, et al. 2014. "Coffee, caffeine, and risk of completed suicide: Results from three prospective cohorts of American adults." The World Journal of Biological Psychiatry. 15(5):377-386.

Ludwig, D.S. and M.I. Friedman. 2014. "Viewpoint Increasing Adiposity, Consequence or Cause of Overeating?" JAMA.311(22):2297-2304.

Lytx. 2014. "Lytx Data Finds Three Dangerous Activities You May Be Doing While Driving Every Day." www.lytx.com/en-us/news-events/press-release/lytx-data-finds-three-dangerous-activities-you-may

Mangeri, F., L. Muntari, G. Forlani, et al. 2014. "A standard ballroom and Latin dance program to improve fitness and adherence to physical activity in individuals with type 2 diabetes and in obesity." Diabetology Metabolic Syndrome 6:74.

Mann, T. A.J. Tomiyama, E. Westling, et al. 2007. "Medicare›s search for effective obesity treatments: diets are not the answer." Am Psychol.62(3):220-33.

Mazzanti, G. L. Battinelli, C. Pompeo, et al. 2008. "Inhibitory activity of Melissa officinalis L. extract on Herpes simplex virus type 2 replication." Nat Prod Res.22(16):1433-40.

McClean P.L., V. Parthsarathy, E. Faivre, C. Holscher. 2011. "The diabetes drug liraglutide prevents degenerative processes in a mouse model of Alzheimer's disease." J Neurosci. 31(17):6587-94.

McNitt-Gray, Ph.D., Jill. 2008. "Anatomy of a Dancer." Dancing with the Stars." Season 7 Week 8 Results Show. November 11, 2008 .

MD Anderson Cancer Center. 2015. "Coriolus versicolor Detailed Scientific Review." www.mdanderson.org/education-and-research/resources-for-professionals/clinical-tools-and-resources/cimer/therapies/herbal-plant-biologic-therapies/coriolus-versicolor-scientific.html

Merritt, MA., I. Tzoulaki, S.S. Tworoger, et al. 2015. "Investigation of Dietary Factors and Endometrial Cancer Risk Using a Nutrient-wide Association Study Approach in the EPIC and Nurses' Health Study (NHS) and NHSII". Cancer Epidemiol Biomarkers Prev. 24(2):466-71.

Miller-Keane Encyclopedia and Dictionary of Medicine, Nursing, and Allied Health, Seventh Edition. S.V. "endorphin." 2016. www.medicaldictionary.thefreedictionary.com/endorphineuroscience

Montgomery, P., A.J. Richardson. 2009. Omega-3 Fatty Acids for Bipolar Disorder (Review)The Cochrane Collaboration. John Wiley & Sons, Ltd.

Morton, W.A., G.G. Stockton. "Methylphenidate Abuse and Psychiatric Side Effects." Prim Care Companion J Clin Psychiatry. 2(5): 159-164.

Mowry, E., A.Hedstrom, M. Gianfrancesco, et al. 2015. "Greater Consumption of Coffee is Associated with Reduced Odds of Multiple Sclerosis." American Academy of Neurology. Platform Session.

Nagano, M.,K. Shimizu, R. Kondo, et al., 2010. Reduction of depression and anxiety by 4 weeks Hericium erinaceus intake.Biomed Res.31(4):231-7.

Nagashima, J., H. Musha, H. Nakada, et al. 2010. "Three-month exercise and weight loss program improves heart rate recovery in obese persons along with cardiopulmonary function." Journal of Cardiology. 56: 79-84.

National Osteoporosis Foundation. 2016. www.nof.org/conditions-and-medicines-that-can-cause-falls/

Natural Revolution. 2015. "List of Countries That Banned Genetically Modified Food." www.naturalrevolution.org/list-countries-banned-genetically-modified-food/

NIA/NIH 2016. www.nia.nih.gov/alzheimers/publication/alzheimers-disease-fact-sheet

NIH (National Institutes of Health). 2013. "Falls and older adults." www.nihseniorhealth.gov/falls/aboutfalls/01.html

NIH. 2016. www.ods.od.nih.gov/factsheets/VitaminB6-HealthProfessional/

NINDS, 2016.

www.ninds.nih.gov/disorders/parkinsons_disease/detail_parkinsons_disease. htm

Olsson, C.J. 2012. "Dancing Combines the Essence for Successful Aging." Frontiers in Aging Neuroscience. 6: 155.

M.P. (Miss P.) 2015. "Will DanceSport Be in the 2020 Olympic Games in Tokyo?" Dance Comp Review. www.dancecompreview.com/will-dancesport-be-in-the-2020-olympic-games-10-reasons-to-consider/

Paffenbarger, Jr., Ralph. 1978. "Harvard Alumni Study. Physical activity as an index of heart attack risk in college alumni." American Journal of Epidemiology. 108 (3) 161-175.

Papakostas, G.I., R.C. Shelton, J.M. Zajecka, et al. 2012. "L-methylfolate as adjunctive therapy for SSRI-resistant major depression: results of two randomized, double-blind, parallel-sequential trials." Am J Psychiatry. 169(12):1267-74.

PubMedPapakostas, G.I., R.C. Shelton, J.M. Zajecka, et al. 2012. "L-methylfolate as adjunctive therapy for SSRI-resistant major depression: results of two randomized, double-blind, parallel-sequential trials." Am J Psychiatry. 169(12): 1267-74

Pinniger, R., R.F. Brown, E.B. Thorsteinsson, P. McKinley. 2012. "Argentine tango dance compared to mindfulness meditation and a waiting-list control: a randomised trial for treating depression." Complement Ther Med. 20(6):377-84

Rahal, M., A.C. Alonso, F.R. Andrusaitis, et al. 2015. "Analysis of static and dynamic balance in healthy elderly practitioners of Tai Chi Chuan versus ballroom dancing." Clinics (3) 01.

Rains, T.M., H.J. Leidy, K.D. Sanoshy, et al. 2015. "A randomized, controlled, crossover trial to assess the acute appetitive and metabolic effects of sausage and egg-based convenience breakfast meals in overweight premenopausal women." Nutr J. 14: 17.

EAiXAP2FPAX11wXAP3DPAXXAP3DPAX&level=3XAP2FPA6J7I3kztATGuYyXAP yXAP2BPAXDahIQXAP3DPAXXAP3DPAX www.sydneysymposium.unsw.edu.au/2001/downloads/LearyDraft2001.doc

Raji, C. RSNA Press Release. 2012. "Active Lifestyle Boosts Brain Structure and Slows Alzheimer's Disease."

Relkin, N. 2014. "Clinical trials of intravenous immunoglobulin for Alzheimer's disease." J Clin Immunol. 2014.34 Suppl 1:S74-9.

Richards, J. 2013. "Mystery of Movement." www.royalsoced.org.uk/cms/files/youngpeople/ Mystery%20of%20Movement/disscussion%202.pdf

Romenets, S.R., J. Anang, S. Fereshtehnejad, et al. 2015. Tango for treatment of motor and non-motor manifestations in Parkinson's disease: A randomized control study. Complementary Therapies in Medicine. 23(2): 175-184.

Ross, G.W., R.D. Abbott, H. Petrovitch, et al. 2000. "Association of Coffee and Caffeine Intake With the Risk of Parkinson Disease Free." JAMA. 283: (20)2674-2679.

Rubio-Tapia, A. J.F. Ludvigsson, T.L, Brantner, et al. 2012. "The prevalence of celiac disease in the United States." Am J Gastroenterology. 107(10): 1538-44.

Sabaratnam, V., K.H. Wong, M. Naidu, et al. 2013. "Neuronal Health – Can Culinary and Medicinal Mushrooms Help?" J Tradit Complement Med. 2013. 3(1): 62–68.

Sahib, S. 2010.American Academy of Neurology. "Can chocolate lower your risk of stroke?" ScienceDaily.www.sciencedaily.com/releases/2010/02/100211163114.htm

Santoro N, Komi J. Prevalence and impact of vaginal symptoms among postmenopausal women. J Sex Med 2009;6:2133-2142.

Scarmeas, N., Y. Stern, M. Tang, et al. 2006. "Mediterranean Diet and Risk for Alzheimer's Disease." Ann Neurol. 59(6): 912-921.

Scarmeas, N. 2009. "Physical Activity, Diet and Risk of Alzheimer's Disease." Journal of the American Medical Association 303:627-237.

Schmit S.L., H. S. Rennert, G. Rennert, S. B. Gruber. 2016. "Coffee Consumption and the Risk of Colorectal Cancer." Cancer Epidemiology Biomarkers & Prevention. 25 (4): 634

Seppälä J, H. Koponen, H. Kautiainen, et al. 2013. "BMC Psychiatry. Association between vitamin b12 levels and melancholic depressive symptoms: a Finnish population-based study." BMC Psychiatry. 24;13:145.

Shapiro, F. 2014. "The Role of Eye Movement Desensitization and Reprocessing (EMDR) Therapy in Medicine: Addressing the Psychological and Physical Symptoms Stemming from Adverse Life Experiences." Perm J. 18(1):71-77.

Shimizu, M., K. Johnson, B. Wansink, et al. 2014. "In good company. The effect of an eating companion's appearance on food intake." Vol 83 263–268.

Shimazu T., M. D. Hirschey, J. Newman, et al. 2012. "Suppression of Oxidative Stress by B-Hydroxybutyrate, an Endogenous Histone Deacetylase Inhibitor." Science, Vol. 339 (6116) 211-214.

Shin, H.W., S.J. Chung. 2012. "Drug-Induced Parkinsonism." J Clin Neurol. 8(1):15-21.

Shurkin J.N 1992. "Terman's Kids: The Groundbreaking Study of How the Gifted Grow Up." Little, Brown & Co. 317 p.

Sian, J. Y. Riederer, M Gerlach. 1999. "MPTP- Induced Parkinsonian Syndrome." Basic Neurochemistry: Molecular, Cellular and Medical Aspects 6th edition.

Singh, G.M., R. Micha, S. Khatibzadeh,et al. 2010. "Estimated Global, Regional, and National Disease Burdens Related to Sugar-Sweetened Beverage Consumption in 2010." Circulation. doi: 10.1161/circulationaha.114.010636

Sinha, M., Y.C. Jang, J. Oh, et al. 2014. "Restoring Systemic GDF11 Levels Reverses Age-Related Dysfunction in Mouse Skeletal Muscle." Science. Vol 344(6184): 649-652.

Smith, B., D.L. Wingard, T.C. Smith, et al. 2006. "Does Coffee Consumption Reduce the Risk of Type 2 Diabetes in Individuals With Impaired Glucose?" Diabetes Care 2006 Nov; 29(11): 2385-2390.

Snowdon, D.A., S.J. Kemper, J.A. Mortimer, et al. 1996. "Linguistic Ability in Early Life and Cognitive Function and Alzheimer's Disease in Late Life Findings From the Nun Study." JAMA. 275(7) 528-532.

Snowdon. D. A. 1997. "Aging and Alzheimer's Disease: Lessons from the Nun Study." The Gerontologist 37(2):150-156.

Sofi,F., F. Cesari, R. Abbate, et al.2008. "Adherence to Mediterranean diet and health status: meta-analysis." BMJ 2008;337:a1344.

Sollitto, Mario. 2016. "6 things that cause the elderly to fall." www.agingcare.com/ Articles/Falls-in-elderly-people-133953.htm

Santoro N, Komi J. Prevalence and impact of vaginal symptoms among postmenopausal women. J Sex Med 2009;6:2133-2142.

Society for Personality and Social Psychology. "Couples who have sex weekly are happiest: More sex may not always make you happier, according to new research." ScienceDaily. ScienceDaily, 18 November 2015. <www.sciencedaily.com/ releases/2015/11/151118101718.htm>.

Sorond, F.A., S. Hurwitz, D.H. Salat, et al. 2013. "Neurovascular coupling, cerebral white matter integrity, and response to cocoa in older people." Neurology 10.1212/ WNL.ob013e3182a351aa

Stulberg, D., B. Ewigman, J. Hickner, et al. 2008. "Antidepressants causing sexual problems? Give her Viagra." J Fam Pract. 57(12): 793–796.

Suez , J. Korem T, Zeevi D, et al. 2014. Artificial sweeteners induce glucose intolerance by altering the gut microbiota. Nature.14:181-186.

Sunni, A.A., R. Latif. 2014. "Effects of chocolate intake on Perceived Stress; a Controlled Clinical Study." Int J Health Sci (Qassim). 8(4): 393-401.

Tahereh, E., Najafi M. 2013. Traditional and Modern Uses of Natural Honey in Human Diseases: A Review. Iran J Basic Med Sci. 16(6): 731–742.

Takahashi K, Okada M, Ozaki T, et al. Safety and efficacy of oestriol for symptoms of natural or surgically induced menopause. Hum Reprod. 2000 May;15(5):1028-36.

Takahashi, M, T. Yamada. 1999. "Viral etiology for Parkinson's disease—a possible role of influenza A virus infection." Jpn J Infect Dis. 52(3): 89-98.

Tan, G., DC Hammond, G. Joseph. 2005. "Hypnosis and irritable bowel syndrome: a review of efficacy and mechanism of action." Am J Clin Hypn. 47(3):161-78.doi: 10.1016/j.lungcan.2009.03.012.

Tang, N., Y. Wu, B. Wang et al. 2010. "Coffee consumption and risk of lung cancer: a meta-analysis." Lung Cancer. 67(1):17-22.

Tartar, B. 2016. "Interview with Powerlifter Jeff Telljohn." www.criticalbench.com/ Jeff-Telljohn.htm

Teixeira, P., E. Carraca, D. Markland, M. Silva, et. al. 2012. Exercise, physical activity, and self-determination theory: A systematic review. Int J Behav Nutr Phys Act. 9:78.

Terry, P., M. Doumas, A.M. Wing. 2009. "Dissociations between motor timing, motor coordination, and time perception after the administration of alcohol or caffeine." Psychopharmacology, (Berl);202:719-29.

Toovey, S., S.S. Jick, C.R. Meier. 2011. "Parkinson's disease or Parkinson symptoms following seasonal influenza." Influenza Other Respir Viruses. 5(5):328-33.

Torkelson, J., E. Sweet, M.R. Martzen, et al. 2012. "Phase 1 Clinical Trial of Trametes versicolor in Women with Breast Cancer." Isrn Oncol. Volume 2012, Article ID 251632, 7 pages.

Triantafillidis, J. K., G. Nasioulas, P.A. Kosmidis. 2009. "Colorectal cancer and inflammatory bowel disease: epidemiology, risk factors, mechanisms of carcinogenesis and prevention strategies." Anticancer Res. 29(7): 2727-37.

Turnbaugh, P.J., R.E. Ley, M.A. Mahowald, et al. 2006. "An obesity-associated gut microbiome with increased capacity for energy harvest." Nature 444, 1027-1031.

Ursano, M.D., C. Bell, M.D.S. Eth, et al. 2010. "Practice Guideline for the Treatment of Patients with Acute Stress Disorder and Posttraumatic Stress Disorder Work Group On ASD and PTSD." www.psychiatryonline.org/pb/assets/raw/sitewide/practice_guidelines/guidelines/acutestressdisorderptsd.pdf

Vaillant, G.E. 2012. Triumphs of Experience: The Men of the Harvard Grant Study. Belknap Press. 480 pages.

Vandeven, N, P. Nghiem. 2012 Complete Spontaneous Regression of Merkel Cell Carcinoma Metastatic to the Liver: Did Lifestyle Modifications and Dietary Supplements Play a Role? Global Advanced Health Medicine. 1(5):22-23.

Veerman, J.L., G.N. Healy, L.J. Cobiac, et al. 2011. "Television viewing time and reduced life expectancy: a life table analysis." Br J Sports Med. 46(13) 927.

Verghese, M.D., R.B. Lipton, M.J. Katz, et al. 2003. "Leisure Activities and the Risk of Dementia in the Elderly." N Engl J Med 348:2508-2516.

Wang, Y., X.J. Liu, L, Robitaille, et al. 2013. "Effects of vitamin C and vitamin D administration on mood and distress in acutely hospitalized patients." American Journal of Clinical Nutrition. 10.3945/ajcn.112.056366

WDSF (World DanceSport Federation) 2016. "Fit Through Dance." www.worlddancesport.org/About/All/Fit_Through_Dance

Weaver, F.M., K.A. Follett, M. Stern. et al. 2012. "Randomized trial of deep brain stimulation for Parkinson disease: Thirty-six-month outcomes." Neurology. 79(1): 55-65.

WHO (World Health Organization). 2016. "Obesity and Overweight Fact Sheet" www.who.int/mediacentre/factsheets/fs311/en/

Willcox D.C., B.J. Willcox, L.W. Poon LW. 2011. "Centenarian studies: important contributors to our understanding of the aging process and longevity." Curr Gerontol Geriatr Res. 2010:1-8.

Williams, S., S. Tamburic, C. Lally. 2009. "Eating chocolate can significantly protect the skin from UV light." J Cosmet Dermatol. 2009 Sep;8(3):169-73.

Willey, Jo. 2014. "Red Meat Is Direct Cause Heart Disease, Experts Warn. Express News." www.express.co.uk/news/uk/531438/Red-meat-cause-heart-disease-link-experts

Wing, R.R., R. W. Jeffrey. 1999. "Benefits of recruiting participants with friends and increasing social support for weight loss and maintenance." J Consult Clin Psychol. 67(1):132-8.

Wolbling RH, K. Leonhardt 1994. "Local therapy of Herpes simplex with dried extract from Melissa officinalis." Phytomedicine. 1:25-31.

Wong, K., M. Naidu, RP David, et.al. 2012. Neuroregenerative potential of Lion's Mane mushroom, Hericium erinaceus (Bull.: Fr.) Pers. (higher Basidiomycetes), in the treatment of peripheral nerve injury (review). International Journal of Medicinal Mushrooms. 14(5):427-46.

Xiaoshuang D., J.M. Stanilka, C. A. Rowe, et al. 2015. "Consuming Lentinula edodes (Shiitake) Mushrooms Daily Improves Human Immunity: A Randomized Dietary Intervention in Healthy Young Adults." Journal of the American College of Nutrition. 34(6):478-487.

Yang, Q. 2010. "Gain Weight by 'Going Diet?' Artificial Sweeteners and the Neurobiology of Sugar Cravings." Yale Journal of Biology and Medicine 83(2): 101-108.

Young, S.N. 2007. "Folate and depression—a neglected problem." J Psychiatry Neurosci. 32(2): 80-82.

Zagursky, E. 2015. "Study finds decreased social anxiety among young adults who eat fermented foods." William and Mary News. www.wm.edu/news/stories/2015/fermented-food-social-anxiety-study123.php

Zhu J.S., G.M.Halpern, K. Jones. 1998. "The scientific rediscovery of an ancient Chinese herbal medicine: Cordyceps sinensis: part I." J Altern Complement Med. 4:289-303.

Zivin, K., H.M. Kim, J.F. McCarthy, et al. 2007. "Suicide Mortality Among Individuals Receiving Treatment for Depression in the Veterans Affairs Health System: Associations with Patient and Treatment Setting Characteristics." Am J Public Health. 97(12): 2193–2198.

Index

A

ADMT 155
Alzheimer's 28-34, 41, 72, 82,
121,122, 124, 178, 180–184,
188, 190–195
Aricept 32
ASCVD Risk Estimator 10
AskMD 5, 175

B

Bacterial overgrowth 23
bioelectrical impedance scale 101
Body Mass Index (BMI) 101
breath test 17
B vitamins 18, 61
B6 61, 185
B12 34, 60, 175

C

Celiac Disease 21
chocolate 15, 19, 69, 71-76, 177,
181–185, 188, 191, 194, 195,
197
coffee 71–74, 104, 185–196,
Cordyceps 79, 80, 197
Cornell University Food and Brand
Lab 107, 108
Cytochrome P450 53

D

depression 12, 18, 19, 21, 31, 41,
52–66, 72, 83, 161, 162, 171,
185–193, 197
DEXA scan 101

E

Eagles 165–, 169, 188
EMDR 18, 56-58, 83, 175, 194
Endorphins 75, 75, 162, 163

F

fish oil 33, 62, 63
Food Action Research Center 102
food allergies 22
fructose intolerance 20

G

GeneSight 53, 175
gluten intolerance 17, 20

H

hydrogen breath test 16

I

IBD 19, 22, 23, 24
inflammatory bowel disease 22,
80, 196
IBS 15–25
irritable bowel syndrome 55
Integrative Medicine, finding a
provider 175

L

lactose intolerance 19
Lion's Mane 79, 82
L-methylfolate 18, 19, 24, 52, 54, 55,
60, 193
longevity 45

M

Maitake 79, 187
meditation 193
Mediterranean diet 13, 32, 33, 46,
66, 112, 188, 195
microbiome 66–68, 78, 196
MTHFR 18, 19, 22, 24, 54, 55, 60,
175
methylenetetrahydrofolate reductase
18, 24, 54
muscular hypertrophy 100, 101

mushrooms 71, 78–83, 186, 189, 194, 197
    Cordyceps 79, 80 197
    Lion's Mane 79, 82
    Maitake 79, 187
    MyCommunity 79
    Turkey Tail 78–81
    Reishi 78–81
    Shiitake 80, 197

N

Namenda 32
NMR lipoprofile 10, 175
Nun Study 122, 195

P

Parkinson's disease 35-38, 41, 124–127, 194-196
Probiotics 20, 24, 67
PTSD 56, 57, 175, 186

R

Reishi 78–81S
SAMe 58
Shiitake 80, 197
Shy Away Dance 151
    shy 152–160
social anxiety (SA) 152–155, 189, 197
social engagement 122

T

T2 Dance Crew 133
TBI 39, 40, 41, 127, 128
    Traumatic brain injury 39
TEID diet 95, 103
telomeres 45
TMAO 10, 13, 175
traumatic brain injury 39
Trimethylamine N-oxide 10
Turkey Tail 78–81

V

Viagra 85, 86, 88, 175, 195
vitamins 17, 18, 21, 24, 32, 34, 47, 52, 54, 55, 59-62, 80, 140, 144, 191, 194, 196, 201
    vitamin C 62
    vitamin D 21, 34, 61, 80, 140, 144, 191, 196
    vitamin E 47
VSL#3 20, 68

W

WDSF 164, 196
World DanceSport Federation 164, 196

Z

Zoloft 59, 144, 162

About THE AUTHORS

Dr. Robin Miller, an established author (*The Smart Woman's Guide to Midlife and Beyond* and *Kids Ask the Doctor*), has gathered the knowledge, insights and anecdotes offered in this book over the course of 33 years of treating patients using the principles of integrative medicine. Board certified in Internal Medicine, she trained with Andrew Weil as an Integrative Medicine Fellow at University of Arizona. She is currently Medical Director of Triune Integrative Medicine, a highly innovative integrative medicine clinic in Medford, Oregon. She blogs regularly for Sharecare.com, an interactive health and wellness website founded in conjunction with Dr. Mehmet Oz, where she serves as Executive Advisory Board member. Robin is also a medical reporter and a regular correspondent for KOBI-5, the NBC affiliate in Southern Oregon.

Dave Kahn is a graduate of UCLA and holds a master's degree from USC. He has taught English for UCLA's Dashew Center for International Students and Scholars, as a volunteer in the US Peace Corps and for Los Angeles Unified School District. He currently teaches at Rogue Community College in Southern Oregon. Dave also is a nationally ranked competitive swing dancer. He has been teaching dance in Oregon for well-over a decade, and he is Director of Southern Oregon Swing, which produces the regional SOswing Newsletter and hosts SOswing Convention, its annual event that brings dancers together from across the country. In addition, his experience and accomplishments in the field of physical fitness as a certified personal trainer and record-holding power-lifter uniquely qualify him to offer the insight of the common-sense, doable weight-loss and fitness solutions offered in this book, the groundbreaking Undiet.